Syndrome W

Syndrome W

A Woman's Guide to Reversing Midlife Weight Gain

Revised Edition

Harriette R. Mogul, M.D., M.P.H.

M. Evans

Lanham · New York · Boulder · Toronto · Plymouth, UK

Published by M. Evans

An imprint of The Rowman & Littlefield Publishing Group, Inc.

4501 Forbes Boulevard, Suite 200, Lanham, Maryland 20706

http://www.rlpgtrade.com

Estover Road, Plymouth PL6 7PY, United Kingdom

Distributed by National Book Network

British Library Cataloguing in Publication Information Available

Library of Congress Cataloging-in-Publication Data

Mogul, Harriette R.
  Syndrome W : a woman's guide to reversing midlife weight gain / Harriette R. Mogul. — Rev. ed.
    p. cm.
  Includes bibliographical references and index.
  ISBN 978-1-59077-161-7 (pbk. : alk. paper) — ISBN 978-1-59077-162-4 (electronic)
  1. Middle-aged women—Health and hygiene. 2. Weight loss. 3. Hormones. I. Title.
  RA778.M685 2010
  613.2'5—dc22

                                                              2010006587

Printed in the United States of America

Dedicated to my phenomenal parents, progeny, partner, and patients for their vision and their voices along the path to Syndrome W.

"Poetry is naming things. . . ."

—Gertrude Stein

CONTENTS

PREFACE

THIS BOOK IS ABOUT all the women I see each day as I go through my day—waiting for my low-fat latte at Starbucks, at the ATM at the local bank, in the locker room at the gym or the reception area at the dentist, while having my hair colored or my nails polished.

Weight is the word. It's definitely the topic of all the women over thirty I meet or greet, at any and every store I visit for any reason, especially when I order food (turkey and veggies at the gourmet grocer, pasta with broccoli and sun-dried tomatoes at the pizzeria, stir-fried veggies and chicken Chinese fare, or fajitas, hold the sour cream and cheese). They suspect that I may know something they don't know, and they stare at me and usually ask if I'm a nutritionist. "No," I respond, and the conversation just evolves from there.

This book is for them, so that when I need to dash out the door after describing what they have (Syndrome W) and what they need for permanent weight loss (The Mogul Protocol: metformin and the Carb-Modified Diet), and they ask, as they inevitably do after this brief interlude, "But, what can I do?" I can now say, "Read my book!"

Acknowledgments

As I think of the many individuals who made this book possible, I understand the length of those Academy Award speeches. Writing *Syndrome W* was the product of many mentors and collaborators, and my thank-you list is a long one.

When you retrain (in a new field) at age fifty, you have to learn quickly. I was fortunate to have had access to a large number of highly experienced basic science researchers and clinicians when I was transitioning back into academic medicine. Special thanks go to Dr. Bernard I. Weinstein, professor of biochemistry; Dr. Stephen R. Gambert, former chairman of the Department of Medicine at New York Medical College, who reviewed our initial data and helped formulate hypotheses about the syndrome; and also A. Louis Southren, chief of the Division of Endocrinology. Other important mentors along the way were Dr. Harold Lebowitz, who first taught me about Syndrome X; Drs. Luciano Rossetti, Harry Shamoon, and Nir Barzilai—at my alma mater, Albert Einstein College of Medicine—who critiqued my initial data in 1996; and their colleague, Dr. Judith Wylie-Rossett at the Diabetes Care Center, and Dr. Leonard Meggs, renowned leaders in diabetes and hypertension and superb physician-scientists.

I'd like to recognize my decade-long research collaborators at Westchester—Dr. Stephen J. Peterson, vice-chairman and professor of clinical medicine; and Dr. Michael Frey, director of our laboratory—for always going that extra mile at the end of some very long days. And I also thank my extramural collaborators Dr. Philip D. K. Lee, professor of pediatrics; and Dr. Barbara Lippe, former director of pediatric endocrinology at UCLA.

My sincere appreciation goes to Dr. William B. Frishman, chairman of medicine, for encouraging me to write *Syndrome W* and reviewing key chapters; Karen Tanenbaum and Lee-Ann Klein for their dedication to our clinical trial participants; Simone Wilker and Lucille D'Agnillo for their ongoing assistance; and Information Services at New York Medical College.

The book would not have been possible without P. J. Dempsey at M. Evans; my talented and energetic editor, Diane Stafford; Mel Berger at the William Morris Agency; Bernadette Ezring from Weil-Gotshal; and the wonderful staff at Manor Vail in Vail, Colorado, and the Rustler in Alta, Utah.

Finally, of course, are my eternal thanks to my extraordinary family: my daughter, Dr. Jennifer Mogul, who never doubted I could complete the book; my son Fred Mogul, a public radio reporter, who read and edited chapters and discussed recipes in between assignments at NPR; my son Douglas B. Mogul, M.D., M.P.H., now a fellow in pediatric gastroenterology at Johns Hopkins and previously a clinical research scholar at the National Institutes of Health, who taught me molecular biology and named Syndrome W; and, most of all, my husband, Malcolm, who yet again postponed his dreams of postretirement travel so that I could realize mine in writing *Syndrome W*.

INTRODUCTION

I Am a Happy Doctor

I'VE HELPED COUNTLESS WOMEN lose weight permanently, regain the waistlines of their youth, and fit into new wardrobes (or very old ones . . . reminders of another life, when they were slimmer and shapelier).

In the past decade, Americans have gotten fatter, but my patients have gotten thinner . . . and healthier. I've heard all their frustration when they first walk in and tell me, "Nothing is working—even the latest and greatest diet and ramping up exercise to five-plus intervals a week!" Then I've witnessed their elation when they review the test results that show conclusively the metabolic cause for the twenty-plus pounds they've gained since their twenties.

It's called Syndrome W, I tell them, and then I get to the best news of all—that this metabolic problem can be reversed with the Mogul Protocol, a combination of a widely used diabetes drug, metformin, along with our Carb-Modified Diet, which act together to reduce the insulin and appetite elevations that are the key players in the progressive weight spiral of Syndrome W sufferers.

My patients are happy, too. They no longer relate to the nightly news reports on the war on obesity—those segments on a revolutionary new diet drug or the celebrity victory over ten pounds in ten days. They smile confidently, watch with detachment, and change the channel. That kind of news doesn't apply to them anymore. They have finally conquered their midlife weight gain. They've worked hard to fit into the clothes they wore before they got Syndrome W, and they have the confidence to know that this time it's forever!

I rejoice in each of their success stories!

As an internist, epidemiologist (clinical researcher), and endocrinologist, I've had an unparalleled opportunity to explore the issues of women and weight gain at the important transitions of adolescence and menopause—a unique chance to talk to and treat hundreds of women at the full spectrum of weight extremes.

Finding Syndrome W was the natural outcome of a career path motivated by a preference for intervention rather than treatment of late-stage disease complications. This was the reason I chose my first job at Student Health Services at Barnard College (the female undergraduate institution of Columbia University in New York City) and why I held the position of director for two decades (1970–1990).

In that era, the mission of college health services changed from Band-Aids to broad-ranged initiatives for promoting health and wellness. My first mandate as health services director was preventing the "freshman ton" (the annual two thousand–pound collective weight gain of the two hundred first-year students) and addressing campus-wide weight problems. In the 1970s, more than half of students entering those hallowed halls on Broadway were overweight or obese. Almost all reported concerns about weight on their health forms.

Notably, at Barnard, I became known more as "the diet doctor" than "the director." It was there (in 1974) that I sought to counter the calorie/carb-loaded dorm fare by developing my Carbohydrate-Modified Diet. This is the diet of the Mogul Protocol, outlined in this book—and it's the same diet I've used for the women, men, and children I've treated for the past thirty-five years! It was there—at Barnard—that I gained valuable insights about why and when women gain weight. And it was there, in an overcrowded conference room, that I first created workshops to help overweight, normal-weight, and underweight women overcome their struggles with the scale.

My interest in obesity research spans five decades. It dates back to a three-month internship when I took care of people with "life-threatening obesity" in my senior year of medical school. The patients had been admitted to the Metabolic Research Unit at Albert Einstein College of Medicine for a large National Institutes of Health–sponsored study to determine the metabolic effects of long-term starvation. I was as surprised then as I am now that nutrition and obesity prevention/treatment aren't parts of the med-school curriculum. Sadly, even today, when the impact of obesity figures prominently in the health and wealth of all Americans, few physicians are taught these skills. Even endocrinologists—we specialists in metabolic disorders—have little expertise and limited knowledge of how to treat the world's most prevalent, preventable, and important metabolic disorder: obesity. Awareness of this gap was one of the main things that spurred me to write this book.

Obesity and eating disorders in women—why women gain weight and why they stray from healthy eating—have also been important areas of focus of my research initiatives. In fact, the systematic data on these common disorders of college women were a major factor in the 1985 creation of the Barnard-Columbia Institute for Medical Research in Women, the first organization devoted entirely to medical research in women in the United States.

These same issues later became an important topic of investigation in a Pew Foundation–funded study that I spearheaded of ten thousand college students. My research in weight gain continued after I shifted gears and moved closer to home to direct the Women's Health Program at New York Medical College and Westchester Medical Center. Even with the broadening of research into acquired and genetic forms of pituitary disease, obesity remains a central theme since virtually all the research participants in these studies are overweight or obese.

My patients tell me that they find me unusually empathetic "for a thin person." They glance at my size 6-ish top and size 10 pants and assume that I have absolutely no familiarity with their issues. But that's not the case. My size in no way reflects my own lifelong weight struggle, overcome only by careful calorie monitoring along with exercise, weight-training, and periods of relaxation.

I do indeed have major obesity genes in my family, and I gained more than a bit of "baby fat" when my tomboy days and athletic build changed and I became a chunky preadolescent after I was forced to restrict my exercise routine due to asthma. In my teen and young adult years, I resumed ballet and team and individual sports and managed to return to my earlier size—12. But even as an unusually active woman, I was never able to consume what's generally considered a normal caloric intake. Early in life, I made peace with my metabolism and my mesomorph body shape.

The truth is, I'm not really thin. I understood, many years ago, that no matter what I did, how little I ate, or how much I exercised, I would never have the body of my slim-hipped, long-legged, cellulite-free classmates at Bryn Mawr. In my thirties, I had to come to grips with the fact that even after five hours of competitive tennis in hundred-plus-degree weather, and even though I sipped Diet Coke, I was never going to be able to wear the same size tennis skirt as my doubles partner, who downed milkshakes.

I learned then that genes ultimately determine our body shapes. They define the limits of where we can go with normal levels of exercise and a reasonable diet. Any attempt to fidget with that equation just won't work.

As we now know, thanks to the research of Dr. Rudy Leibel at Columbia and others, each of us has a predetermined weight set-point—a range of just a few pounds that, like eye color or our blood type, is uniquely our own. It's set in stone for life. Physiologically primed for childbearing, real women do have curves. Only a handful of us are destined to be willowy movie star Gwyneth Paltrows or model-thin Paris Hiltons. Only extreme and dangerous acts such as severe anorexia or bulimic behaviors—what I call "under-nutrition" and "excessive eliminating behaviors"—can alter the equation of your set-point. So don't even think about it.

Unlike most of you reading this book, I don't have Syndrome W. I am that classic pear: smallish waist, larger hips, 34-28-38 at present (although I've been 36-28-40 at times). I will never be thin, and I don't need to be. I got on course with my weight in my fifties when I went on the Carb-Modified Diet after my third child left for college and I had more time and fewer family objections to eating vegetable-based, low-fat protein meals that are the mainstay of this diet. I hit my stride at sixty, accepted my size-12 hips, and began to work out in earnest (three times a week) with a trainer so that I could become a fit pear. I also added nightly dance routines and half-hour lunchtime walks. For me, there's no going back.

So, although I don't have Syndrome W, I can fully relate to the frustration you and other Syndrome W women encounter as midlife weight gain accelerates out of control despite all your best efforts. That's the driving force behind this book—the many hours of data analysis, grant applications, and now thousands of conversations with women of all ages and ethnic groups who, like you, have tried so hard to stem that upward weight spiral that started in perimenopause (or earlier).

Here is everything you need to know so that you, too, can join the ranks of women who have succeeded in losing weight by finding Syndrome W and incorporating the Mogul Protocol into their lives.

Syndrome
W

Part I

YOUR QUESTION:
What's Happened to My Body?

GAINING WEIGHT AND LOSING YOUR WAIST aren't exactly "aging benefits," but those were the two very obvious things that happened when you turned forty—or shortly thereafter. And when you tried all your old tricks for taking off a few pounds, suddenly nothing seemed to work. You developed a strong hunch that something was wrong with your metabolism, but answers were hard to come by. Then, you heard about something called "Syndrome W," and a book on that subject that's becoming so revolutionary and results oriented that now even doctors are recommending it.

So here you are. You want to find out whether Syndrome W could be the reason for your weight escalation. Here's the plan: review the symptoms and stories in the book and see whether you can relate to them. Then check this out with your doctor to get the gold standard glucose-tolerance test that tells whether you have Syndrome W. Fortunately, more and more primary care physicians are becoming aware of Syndrome W and will work with you to find and fix it!

In part I you'll learn all about Syndrome W. Armed with answers to the mystery of midlife weight gain, you, too, can join the ranks of our patients and countless other women who lose weight and gain health with the Mogul Protocol. Even if you find out you're one of the fortunate few forty-somethings without Syndrome W, the Carb-Modified Diet and other easily-adopted strategies in the book will work well to help you shed those unwanted extra pounds painlessly and permanently.

Read on!

Chapter 1

WAIST (NOT)

Gaining Weight and Losing Your Waist?

"NOTHING WORKS! I used to have a waistline and wear a size five. I always ate healthy and exercised regularly and never had any problem losing weight. Now, no matter what I do, I just can't get rid of the extra twenty-plus pounds I've gained since my twenties. Even when I work out every day, the scale doesn't budge. None of the diets that work for everyone else makes any difference at all for me. Even those new low-carb plans stop working the minute I go past phase I—the superstrict, eat-no-carb part that I could never live on for life, anyway. Then, if I finally manage to lose a few pounds on South Beach or Atkins, I'm back up the minute I add a few fruits or a healthy, high-fiber (good) carb or any variety to my diet!"

"Everything changed the day I woke up on my fortieth birthday. I swear, it's like a switch went off. Now I don't even recognize my reflection in full-length mirrors or the glass windows I pass on the streets. I just can't understand what's happening to my body."

"Clothes are another big issue. I've already given away all those form-fitting outfits I used to love to wear, and now I don't buy anything with a belt. Luckily, fashions for the 'mature' woman today come in nice fabrics, neutral colors, and pretty prints that I can wear to work and when I go out. Thank goodness for those elastic waists in pants that expand under loose-fitting tops and straight-cut jackets. They go a long way toward camouflaging the extra inches I'm adding to my waist each year. But it's getting harder and harder to find clothes that fit! What's wrong?"

I'm sure you recall a time when you rarely worried about what you ate and you maintained your weight simply by consuming mostly healthy foods and doing some exercise. A few extra pounds caused little chagrin because you had no problem taking them off. But that was *before* the radical detour your body took after your thirties. And living with the extra pounds you've packed on has been anything but fun.

Desperately Seeking Slender

The hardest part is that you've completely lost your waist. That very elusive "narrowest circumference between the bottom of the breastbone and the top of the pelvic bone" is gone! You have to admit it: you're basically shaped like an egg, or a woman in her fifth month of pregnancy, or (worse) Humpty Dumpty.

Surely, your body can't betray you, but at times it seems that's exactly what has happened. You just can't win. It's a battle of the fittest, and you're losing. And you feel increasingly frustrated, angry, sad, and hopeless.

Outsourcing: Off to the Doctor

Today's savvy thinking woman always looks for answers, so of course you don't just languish in your sorrow, whining about this unwelcome weight gain. Instead, you take a proactive approach. You just need some help here—a logical explanation for this progressive, never-ending weight spiral.

Off you go to your doctor to get some lab tests to find the cause of this new and mysterious metabolic problem. When all the tests come back in normal range, you're told that you're probably off in your calculation—eating more and exercising less than you think. You're advised to "Exercise more! Eat less!" Sometimes the diet you're given has more food on it than you're eating each day.

Sadly, many doctors remain convinced that you're underestimating the calories you consume each day and overestimating the number of miles you walk or the number of hours in aerobics classes or gym workouts. If, despite the newly accumulated pounds, you're not very overweight, you may even be told, "All women gain weight as they age. So be less neurotic and just accept those extra pounds gracefully!"

What If? How about a Metabolic Makeover?

How about a metabolic makeover? A chance to return to earlier, carefree days when the scale was friendlier, more like what you'd come to expect when you dieted and exercised regularly? **What if you took a new and *different* set of lab tests and got some good news for a change? What if you found out, "Yes, you really *do* have an abnormality in your metabolism—and it's called Syndrome W?"** It's why, despite all your best efforts, none of the diets—even the newest and lowest low-carbohydrate ones—work. What if I added two more important details:

- This type of metabolic shift is completely correctable.
- It can be fixed *forever* by taking a safe, inexpensive, and widely used medication along with an easy-to-follow, superhealthy, enjoyable, nondeprivation diet that work together to treat the cause of the problem.

I bet you'd stop in your tracks at the idea that your weight escalation could have a cause and a cure. Then, if you're like any of the many women I've treated successfully over the years, you'd smile widely and rejoice. Hallelujah, you've finally found Syndrome W!

Chapter 2

SYNDROME W: WHAT'S IN A NAME?

We Hear a Familiar Refrain . . .

THAT WAS YOUR STORY. HERE'S MINE.

My patients all tell the same story; in fact, the message is so consistent that I can narrate it for new patients of a certain age and a certain shape as they walk into my office, even before they tell me why they've come. Their astonishment as I list the details of their medical histories is indescribable. Their eyes widen, and they nod their heads in disbelief as I summarize their decade-long weight struggle, their daily pilgrimages to the health club, and their need to enlarge their closets to accommodate an array of increasingly sized skirts and pants due to their unwillingness to dispose of older and costlier clothes.

They quickly grasp the truth—that the story of Syndrome W is a common reality of most midlife women. It doesn't discriminate. It doesn't matter where you were born, how well you were educated, or what you do for a living. You can have all the symptoms of Syndrome W, and you can live with it for many years without a diagnosis.

Most of the women I see, like you, suspect correctly that something must be wrong. They search vainly for an explanation for this dramatic change in body shape after a lifetime of relatively normal weight regulation. They are intelligent and motivated seasoned dieters with active lifestyles, and they all know a lot about nutrition. They understand that decreased caloric intake combined with increased exercise is supposed to produce weight loss. So they rev up their activity level, working out many hours a week. All valiantly attempt to restrict their calories, trying every diet in succession—all to no avail. Time to look elsewhere, talk to others who might know more.

Same Song, 442nd Verse

This is the chronicle I've heard over and over again from hundreds of women who were trying hard to change their bodies and getting nothing back from their efforts. Here are the puzzling stats from my first publication:

- More than 90 percent of the first three hundred women we saw exercised three or more times a week for forty-five minutes or more at each exercise session.
- Some worked out an hour a day at local gyms.
- Two ran thirty to forty miles each week, and one mountain-biked fifty miles every weekend.
- Two were aerobics instructors, clocking in twenty hours of high-intensity exercise weekly.

How absurd to blame lack of exercise or so-called sedentary lifestyle for the profound midlife weight gain in these women! There had to be a different explanation. It was the analysis of these data that made all of us in our menopausal health program shake our heads and speculate that something had to be going on to account for all of the overweight women whose lifestyles were well aligned with public health guidelines. That's what drove us to look harder for a hormonal cause for that all-too-common midlife weight gain and what helped us, ultimately, find and define the underlying metabolic defect—Syndrome W.

Why It's Called Syndrome W

I'm sure you're wondering why we call it "Syndrome W."

Syndrome **W** represents a cluster of clinical components that start to appear as women begin to experience the earliest symptoms of menopause, a period called perimenopause. The syndrome's name captures its key elements:

- **W**eight gain
- **W**aist gain

- White-coat hypertension (blood pressure elevations at the doctor's office)
- in **W**omen

One additional symptom is a universal feature of Syndrome W, and that's a dramatic increase in appetite or the development of new food cravings, especially for sweets and carbohydrates. For most midlife women who ate normally before, this can lead to out-of-control (or binge) eating.

If you have Syndrome **W**, you may find that when you take "just a taste" of the sugar-laced, "low-fat" foods that have proliferated in the past decade, you're unable to stop after just one Oreo or a forkful of fudge cake. This makes it a lot harder to stick to a diet and lose those newly accumulated pounds.

We used the name Syndrome W for another reason. Syndrome W is an early form (and alphabetical precursor) of another, more advanced clinical condition that was originally termed Syndrome **X** (now known as "the metabolic syndrome"—see chapter 13). Both disorders are caused by a metabolic disturbance called "insulin resistance."

The hallmark of Syndrome W is an elevation in insulin levels in the bloodstream (hyperinsulinemia) without the characteristic blood sugar abnormalities that define type 2 diabetes. So if you have Syndrome W, you not only have a metabolic defect, you have a culprit and a cause for your weight gain that's real, not imagined.

But the best part is the happy ending to the Syndrome W story. Syndrome W is not only detectable—it's also completely correctable. You no longer have to tolerate and live with the weight spiral that's the recurring theme of forty- and even thirty-something overweight women. With the Mogul Protocol, our two-pronged program, this midlife malady can be reversed. The earlier you find it, the easier it is to fix Syndrome W. So let's get started.

Chapter 3

YOUR SYNDROME W STORY

Have You Gained Twenty Pounds Since Your Twenties?

A DECADE AGO WHEN WE FIRST identified Syndrome W, that was the first question we asked, and it still is. If your answer is yes and you're having trouble losing weight, see whether the list below speaks to you. If you can relate to three or more of the following, you may have Syndrome W.

You:

- Were thin or normal weight during your childhood and young adult years.
- Wore a size three to thirteen.
- Maintained your weight easily for most of your adult life.
- Took off extra pounds easily by eating right, dieting intermittently, exercising, and staying active.
- Started to pack on pounds at age forty, when your weight began to escalate inexplicably and your usual weight-loss strategies failed.
- Watched unwanted pounds accumulate.
- Saw your size sixes become size eights, then tens and twelves.
- Experienced a waist-diameter surge that resulted in a change in contour (you went from hourglass to egg).
- Noticed a back-view silhouette unchanged from your twenties and thirties but a profile that resembled a woman in the middle trimester of pregnancy.
- Wound up a post-forty woman who looked four months pregnant perennially.

Your SWS (Syndrome W Score) Calls for an SOS

Now let's get specific and calculate your Syndrome W score using questions from the questionnaire I still send to all new patients. Answer the following questions and then total your score:

The Syndrome W Scale

Check yes or no.

1. Has the weight gain been mostly at your waist rather than below your waist (in your hips and butt) or all over (on your entire frame, hips, thighs, back, and arms)? Yes ☐ No ☐
2. Has your belt size increased by two inches or more since you were thirty? Yes ☐ No ☐
3. Have you had a two-size increase in your skirt or pants since your thirties? Yes ☐ No ☐
4. Do you have a noticeable increase in appetite? Yes ☐ No ☐
5. Do you have intense food cravings, especially for sweets or carbs, and does this make you overeat or binge? Yes ☐ No ☐
6. Although you can easily skip meals, do you find that once you start to eat, you find yourself getting hungrier and eating large quantities? Yes ☐ No ☐
7. Do you think you eat more than you used to? Yes ☐ No ☐
8. Do you follow a low-fat, high-carbohydrate diet? Yes ☐ No ☐
9. Have you ever lost weight with a high-protein, low-carbohydrate diet? Yes ☐ No ☐
10. Have you decreased your exercise level in the past six to twelve months? Yes ☐ No ☐
11. Do you find that you eat less or exercise more and are still unable to lose weight? Yes ☐ No ☐
12. Is stress at home or at work contributing to your weight gain? Yes ☐ No ☐
13. Do you think your weight gain was associated with any medication or hormone replacement? Yes ☐ No ☐
14. Was your blood pressure higher than usual when you last went in to see your doctor even though you have always had low or normal blood pressure? Yes ☐ No ☐
15. Is your HDL (good cholesterol) less than 50? Yes ☐ No ☐

To calculate your score, add one point for each "yes" on questions 1–6 and 11, 14, and 15, and each "no" for 10, 12, and 13. (Questions 7–9 are not included in the tally.)

If your score is 6 or more *or* if your lifetime weight pattern resembles the following imprint, you probably have Syndrome W.

5. Do you currently consider yourself overweight?	●Yes	○No
6. Have you ever been more than 20 pounds overweight?	●Yes	○No
7. Have you gained 20 pounds or more since your twenties?	●Yes	○No
8. Do you currently restrict calories for weight reduction or maintenance?	●Yes	○No
9. Did you gain weight with menopause (menopausal women only)?	●Yes	○No

10. IF YOU ANSWERED "Yes" TO QUESTIONS 6, 7, 8 OR 9, PLEASE COMPLETE:

1) Has your weight gain been predominantly at the waist rather than all over?	●Yes	○No
2) Has your belt-size increased by 2 inches or more since age 30?	●Yes	○No
3) Have you had a 2-size increase in skirt or pants size since your 30's (e.g. size 10 to 14)?	●Yes	○No
4) Have you had a detectable increase in appetite?	●Yes	○No
5) Do you have intense food cravings (e.g. for sweet foods) that cause you to overeat or binge?	●Yes	○No
6) Do you find that although you can easily skip meals, once you start to eat you find yourself getting "hungrier", eating large quantities or "binging"?	●Yes	○No
7) Do you think you eat more than you used to eat?	○Yes	●No
8) Do you follow a "low-fat, high carbohydrate diet"?	●Yes	○No
9) Have you ever lost weight with a high protein, low carbohydrate diet?	●Yes	○No
10) Have you decreased your exercise level in the past 6 - 12 months?	○Yes	●No
11) Do you find you eat less or exercise more and are still unable to lose weight?	●Yes	○No
12) Do you think stress either at home or on the job is contributing to weight gain?	○Yes	●No
13) Do you think your weight gain was associated with any medication or hormone?	○Yes	●No

11. Please describe your lifetime weight history:

1) Were you a thin-normal weight child?	●Yes	○No
2) Were you a thin-normal weight adult?	●Yes	○No
3) Were you normal-slightly overweight most of your life?	○Yes	●No
4) Did you struggle with weight most of your life?	○Yes	●No
5) Did you gain 20 pounds or more (that you were unable to lose) after a pregnancy?	○Yes	●No

12. Please indicate the average size range in each age group.

Women

pants, skirt or dress size	[< 6]	[6 - 8]	[8 - 10]	[10 - 12]	[12 - 14]	[14 - 16]	[16 - 18]	[> 18]
Teenage (<21)	○	●	○	○	○	○	○	○
Young Adult (21 - 30)	○	○	●	○	○	○	○	○
Adult (>30)	○	○	○	○	○	●	○	○

Men

pants size (inches)	[< 32]	[32 - 34]	[34 - 36]	[36 - 38]	[38 - 40]	[40 - 50]	[> 50]
Teenage (<21)	○	●	○	○	○	○	○
Young Adult (21 - 30)	○	○	○	●	○	○	○
Adult (>30)	○	○	○	○	○	●	○

PLEASE DO NOT WRITE IN THIS AREA

[SERIAL]

Connecting the Dots

Trends in Clothing Sizes at Various Ages

Women's pants, skirt, dress size	<6	6–8	8–10	10–12	12–14	14–16	16–18	>18
Teen		X						
Young adult 21–30				X				
Adult >30						X		

(continued)

Men's pants size (inches)	<32	32–34	34–36	36–38	38–40	40–50	>50
Teen		X					
Young adult 21–30				X			
Adult >30						X	

Weighing Your "W" Potential

Two additional questions help clarify your chance of having Syndrome W.

1. Was your blood pressure higher than usual when you went to a doctor's office (after a lifetime of normal or even low blood pressure)?
2. Is your HDL (the good cholesterol) less than 50?

I use the last two questions to shortcut the screening in social settings when I'm asked, "How can I tell whether I (or my wife or my sister) have Syndrome W?" Clearly, there's no way to reconstruct the Syndrome W symptom checklist in the confines of a normal conversation. In studies using sophisticated computer models, either a single blood pressure greater than 140/85 (in a doctor's office) *or* an HDL less than 50 (in women with no known diabetes) correctly predicted more than four out of five women with Syndrome W.

If the Belt Fits . . .

If you've seen yourself on these pages (so far), you're undoubtedly excited that a solution could be close at hand. You're probably wondering what you need to do next to find out whether Syndrome W is part of your weight-gain story. You have just a few final steps before starting the Mogul Protocol and experiencing the joy of other women who've reversed midlife weight gain forever.

Chapter 4

FINDING YOUR SYNDROME W DOCTOR

Lining Up an Ally for Your Weight-Loss Quest

NOW YOU'RE READY TO GET your weight-loss plan in gear.

First you need to find a physician to order the necessary lab tests to determine whether you have Syndrome W. Even with all the evidence in favor of the diagnosis, you need to confirm that you have the characteristic insulin abnormalities before you can go any further. Getting a physician on board from the start is critical to your success. The Mogul Protocol requires adding doctor-prescribed and -monitored medication to the mix of healthy diet and (for some) behavioral change.

Partnering Up

Metformin is a unique and innovative part of the Mogul Protocol that accounts for its high success rate and sets this book apart from all others of the diet genre. So your first task is to find a physician who will listen and respond to you. After you locate the right health-care provider, getting metformin should not be a problem.

Before you request the tests for Syndrome W, make sure you're working with a physician willing to help you get with the program. You need a physician to order the tests for Syndrome W and be comfortable prescribing and monitoring the metformin that's a critical component of your treatment plan.

The Right Doctor for the Right Time

Fortunately, more and more physicians are becoming aware of Syndrome W as a distinct clinical entity. After a decade of preaching the importance of early diagnosis of insulin resistance, it's exciting to see that an increasing number of medical practitioners are now ordering the definitive diagnostic test. If your primary care doctor isn't familiar with Syndrome W, you may need to suggest that he or she go online and access the medical literature databases Medline and PubMed to review our research publications on the signs, symptoms, and treatment of Syndrome W. Medical articles can also be downloaded from our website, www.SyndromeW.com or retrieved from Google.

Virtually all doctors today are all too familiar with the ravages of insulin resistance and encounter manifestations of diabetes and the metabolic syndrome every day in their practices. Many prescribe metformin to treat blood sugar abnormalities in patients with diabetes. An increasing number of practitioners are even using metformin, along with other lifestyle modifications, to prevent diabetes in patients with "prediabetes"—defined now as a fasting blood sugar greater than 99 or a two-hour test greater than 139.

Many primary care physicians also appreciate the advantage of tracking and treating Syndrome W in overweight women with abnormal insulin response curves and incipient blood pressure and lipid abnormalities. Some physicians already use metformin to treat a common disorder of hyperinsulinemia in younger women—polycystic ovarian syndrome (PCOS)—in which similar insulin elevations occur with normal blood sugars.

Most physicians are only too happy to have an obesity treatment that's effective and acceptable to their patients because the current FDA-approved medications—Xenical and Meridia—have major problems (unpleasant side effects). Medication as the cornerstone of a weight-loss program isn't a new concept to the medical community. In fact, ever since 1996, when the National Institutes of Health issued public health guidelines advocating the use of medication as "an adjunct" to diet and exercise and other lifestyle interventions in the treatment of obesity, physicians have increasingly accepted that medication may be necessary to reverse the obesity epidemic.

You want your doctor to have a full understanding of Syndrome W because in the past, diagnosis of this disorder was often delayed due to the fact that Syndrome W women classically have completely normal

blood sugar tests. If you have Syndrome W, getting this diagnosed early and treated early is extremely important because women with Syndrome W may be on the way to bigger problems like diabetes and/or Syndrome X, now called the metabolic syndrome (see chapter 13).

When you first go in to discuss unexpected weight gain with your doctor, while you're still in your forties, you probably don't yet meet the criteria for Syndrome X (especially if you're a careful eater and regular exerciser). Remember that weight gain at the onset of perimenopause may be the first sign or "flag" of insulin resistance. So it's only after you "progress" farther down the insulin pathway that you will see full-fledged abnormalities develop as Syndrome W becomes Syndrome X. I consider Syndrome W the premetabolic syndrome—a warning sign of bigger troubles ahead if you don't nip Syndrome W in the bud.

Moving Right Along

If your internist or family practice doctor remains unconvinced that you have a problem, go see your gynecologist, who has heard hundreds of women ask for weight-loss solutions. Also, because gynecologists already use metformin to treat women with PCOS, they're comfortable with the idea of prescribing it to an older generation of nondiabetic, hyperinsulinemic women.

You can also see an endocrinologist, who will have extensive training in diabetes management. Endocrinologists are quite familiar with all aspects of prescribing metformin, and most have become nutrition-savvy in their years of taking care of people with diabetes.

What you're looking for in a Syndrome W doctor is a physician who will:

- Test you for Syndrome W.
- Supervise your Syndrome W treatment plan, which we call the Mogul Protocol.
- Be willing to prescribe the medication metformin unless you have a health condition that makes it inappropriate for you.

If you've gained twenty pounds since your twenties, fit the profile of Syndrome W, and have been unable to lose weight after six months of attempted lifestyle change that includes regular exercise and calorie restriction, you really need your physician to order additional tests.

Otherwise, you may need to find a new and more responsive physician. (As a case in point, last year I saw a nineteen-year-old who was referred to me because she had gained fifty pounds in five years. Her mother, a medical social worker, had spent ten thousand dollars seeing doctor after doctor at New York's best academic centers, and *no one* ordered insulin levels or found her diagnosis of PCOS.) The urgency of a correct diagnosis can't be emphasized enough!

Chapter 5

GOING FOR THE GOLD (STANDARD TEST)

Getting the Right Test Done the Right Way

TESTING IS NECESSARY to detect the hallmark of Syndrome W—hyper-insulinemia, elevated insulin levels after the performance of a glucose tolerance test. Don't expect your doctor to find these abnormally high insulin levels during a routine health evaluation. They remain undetected in most women with Syndrome W because **most physicians in the United States don't measure insulin levels—not even in patients at high risk for insulin resistance or for type 2 diabetes.**

You may wonder (and rightly so) why no one has caught your problem before now. After all, you go in for routine checkups. You get a Pap smear, breast exam, blood pressure measurement, and urine analysis on a regular basis. You may have a complete physical and some "screening" blood tests to check your risks for developing diabetes or heart disease. But—and this is a big *but*—even if you have Syndrome W, you won't know that anything's wrong with your metabolism because the tests that your doctor orders will be normal. *That's* the tricky part.

Sadly, this kind of rosy assessment only gives you false security. You'll remain unaware of your dysfunctional metabolism, and you may not know that discovering and treating insulin resistance in its early stages—before you develop the blood sugar abnormalities that define diabetes—is the best way to prevent its progression.

Getting Tested

To find out whether you have Syndrome W, your doctor will need to order a glucose tolerance test (GTT) *with* insulin levels (also called an insulin response curve). This is the test that's known in the world of medicine as the gold standard—the kind of test that most reliably diagnoses a suspected medical condition—in this case, Syndrome W. It's like the culture your doctor orders for a urinary tract infection or a biopsy for breast cancer. Confirmation of a diagnosis always requires the gold standard test.

In the case of Syndrome W, the two-hour glucose tolerance test (GTT) *with* insulin levels is the gold standard. During this type of GTT, blood samples are taken for *both* glucose (sugar) and insulin at four points over a two-hour period: fasting, and 30, 60, and 120 minutes after rapidly swallowing a glucose solution with 75 grams of glucose.

Two other versions of the GTT sometimes used are:

1. The 50-gram GTT that's given to pregnant women to detect diabetes during pregnancy.
2. The three-hour GTT to test for hypoglycemia (blood is drawn hourly for three hours after taking glucose).

It's important to note that *neither* of the above should be used to diagnose Syndrome W!

Also, remember that you can't do this evaluation *without* a doctor. **A physician must order your GTT and make sure that it's done according to the following instructions so that the test results can be interpreted accurately.**

Photocopy this page and take it in to show your doctor when you request the test. You will need to emphasize that the test must be done "according to this sheet of instructions" to yield valid information for diagnosing Syndrome W. Then bring the sheet to the laboratory to make sure they draw the blood samples correctly as well.

Instructions for the Two-Hour Glucose Tolerance Test

1. ***Do not*** **restrict carbohydrates (starches) or sugars for three days prior to the test.**

Long-term **strict** adherence to a **very-low-carbohydrate diet** (several months or more) prior to the performance of the test could "normalize" the test results in individuals with mild or "borderline" insulin defects. Discontinue such dietary practices for two weeks prior to testing.

2. **Fast after midnight.**
Take any medications you customarily take, but you should eat or drink nothing except plain water. (This means no coffee or tea.)

3. **Do not participate in strenuous exercise (such as an early morning run or exercise class) the day of your test.**
Exercise improves your "glucose disposal" (how well the cells in your body take up glucose). This will lower the blood sugars measured in the test. If you exercise during the test, you may not get an accurate GTT.

4. **Bring food and fruit juice for after the test**—Please bring along a piece of fruit or a container of orange or apple juice and a protein snack (like cheese or a hardboiled egg) and eat these in the lab before you depart. If you have high insulin levels in the early part of the test, these may cause a dip in your blood sugars later on. Therefore, you need to have just a bit of sugar and some protein after that last blood is drawn to avoid any weakness or dizziness following the test.

Instructions for the Laboratory

Please understand that the purpose of this test is to obtain insulin levels in addition to the glucose levels that are usually drawn for a glucose tolerance test (GTT).

1. Draw fasting glucose and insulin (**two separate tubes**).
2. Administer 75 grams of Glucola with ice and lemon (if available) and advise the patient to drink it as quickly as possible.
3. Draw **two tubes of blood**—one for glucose **and one for insulin** at the following times: 30, 60, and 120 minutes.
4. Please ask the patient to sit quietly during the entire two hours of the test.
5. Make sure the patient eats a snack before she leaves the lab.

Now that you've had your test, your next step is making sure that your test results are interpreted accurately.

Chapter 6

FORMULAS FOR MOVING FORWARD

Getting the Right Take on Your Metabolism

AFTER YOU HAVE the two-hour glucose tolerance and insulin test, the next step is ensuring that you get an accurate interpretation of the findings. All primary care physicians know the American Diabetes Association guidelines for evaluating glucose curves. However, it's not unusual for physicians to contact our office requesting guidelines for calculating and interpreting the insulin response curve. Here's the formula we use:

Insulin Response Curve Formula

Insulin Response Curve = .25 × the fasting insulin +
.5 × the 30-minute insulin + .75 × the 60-minute insulin +
.5 × the 120-minute insulin

Example: fasting = 12, 30-minute = 50,
60-minute = 100, 120-minute = 60

Insulin Response Curve = .25(12) + .5(50) +
.75(100) + .5 (30) = 118

No absolute cutoff value *defines* an abnormal insulin response curve. Similar to the cases of blood sugar, blood pressure, and cholesterol, a continuum exists in which "abnormal" is defined arbitrarily by a consensus of experts. We use 100 (or more) to indicate the presence of hyperinsulinemia. This cutoff is based on the standard used in many research studies. Other insulin values from the GTT that suggest insulin abnormality are:

- A single insulin value higher than 50 at any time in the test
- A fasting level higher than 12

Screen Testing

Is there a simpler way to diagnose Syndrome W? Confirmation of the diagnosis of Syndrome W ultimately requires the gold standard GTT and insulin response curve described above. But there is one reliable screening test that can assess who *is* (and who is not) likely to have Syndrome W—the IGFBP-1. (IGF-binding protein-1 is an obscure protein that circulates in your bloodstream.) Your doctor can use this test to see whether you're a candidate for further testing with a GTT. If you are twenty to forty pounds overweight, you've had a recent fasting blood sugar that's normal (80–100), and you're not taking any steroid medications (for asthma or arthritis), IGFBP-1 is a highly sensitive and highly specific marker of long-term hyperinsulinemia.

Maybe you've heard of a hemoglobin A1C—a simple blood test of long-term or "integrated" blood sugar that enables doctors to spot diabetes in suspect patients and monitor diabetes management in others. Just like A1C is a measure of long-term or "integrated" glucose in the blood, IGFBP-1 is a marker of long-term or "integrated" insulin in the blood.

The production of IGFBP-1 (in the liver) is severely reduced by the high insulin levels of Syndrome W. That's why it's such a good marker of long-term insulin production by the pancreas. An IGFBP-1 with a value less than 10 (collected in the morning before you have eaten breakfast) predicts 100 percent of overweight to mildly obese women with abnormal insulin response curves. It reliably separates the women with and without Syndrome W.

Our research on IGFBP-1 was highlighted (in 1999) for nonmedical audiences in *American Health Magazine*, "Healthy Heart Guide, Life-Saving Breakthroughs," where its description led the list in the article "Ten State-of-the-Heart Discoveries You Need to Know about Now." The usefulness of IGFBP-1 as a simple serum marker for hyperinsulinemia and insulin resistance has been demonstrated in many studies of diverse populations.

IGFBP-1 is increased when sugars become abnormal. (It can even be used to check for blood sugar abnormalities in children with classic type 1 diabetes.) Since IGFBP-1 goes down with insulin excess and goes up with glucose excess, it's an excellent test to distinguish people with Syndrome W, who have abnormal insulin curves, from those with Syndrome X, who also have abnormal glucose curves (see chapter 13). That's why it's ideal for spotting Syndrome W early on, when it's most treatable.

If you're a candidate for the test (see the requirements listed below) and want to learn more about your insulin status without undergoing a two-hour GTT, ask your physician to order an IGFBP-1.

IGFBP-1 is now available in several commercial laboratories, but keep in mind that the accuracy of the results depends on the quality of the laboratory. Several research labs now have commercial divisions that perform the test correctly; two we recommend are Esoterix and Nichols. When you have your blood drawn, make sure that it's sent to one of these two research-oriented labs. (Most commercial laboratories that doctors use send samples to one of them.)

Remember, for your test to be interpreted correctly, the test should be taken first thing in the morning, before you eat anything or engage in any rigorous exercise, because IGFBP-1 goes down after eating and goes up with exercise. It can also go up after prolonged fasting, starvation, or severe caloric restriction (e.g., it is elevated in women with anorexia nervosa).

The IGFBP-1 test is reliable if you:

- Are overweight or mildly obese.
- Are not a diabetic (IGFBP-1 is increased in patients with blood sugar elevations).
- Are not taking steroid medications (these can raise IGFBP-1).
- Are not engaging in fasting for dietary or other reasons (IGFBP-1 goes up if you fast for more than a day or severely restrict caloric intake for several days).

We don't measure fasting insulin alone because IGFBP-1 is a better predictor. Here's why:

- Some people with Syndrome W have elevated insulin response curves but still have a fasting insulin in normal range, especially in the early stages of Syndrome W.

- Experts in diabetes and insulin resistance do not agree on what constitutes a "normal" versus an "abnormal" fasting insulin. Some researchers consider a fasting insulin level above 12 suggestive of an underlying insulin abnormality, but controversy still runs rampant!

Ready to Roll

So now you know everything you need to know to diagnose Syndrome W. At this point you should be "all systems go." You should know how to find a physician and undergo the necessary testing, and along with some help from your doctor, you should be all set to move to the Mogul Protocol. The pages that follow give you more insight about Syndrome W and all the information you need to fix it and stay healthy forever. Create your own unique template for corrective interventions for weight loss based on strategies that have worked for hundreds of Syndrome W women just like you. It's all here, finally in one volume—a manual for change based on a multifaceted approach to long-term weight loss that's data driven, a work in progress that's evolved over a lifetime of helping women (and men and children) reverse their upward weight spiral to become thinner, trimmer, healthier, and happier.

Now it's your turn.

Chapter 7

DECONSTRUCTING THE SYNDROME W CYCLE

A Cautionary Tale

UNFORTUNATELY, you need to know that you can't *just live with* Syndrome W.

Syndrome W is more than just midlife weight gain—it's a red flag, a harbinger of things to come. As described in chapter 2, Syndrome W is an early stage of a serious and significant metabolic disorder—the underlying disturbance in type 2 diabetes, called "insulin resistance." Unchecked, it will undoubtedly lead to diabetes. Almost all women who eventually develop diabetes have passed through this phase.

Second, Syndrome W doesn't stand still. It just silently marches on. Syndrome W signals the start of a vicious and progressive cycle of weight gain → insulin resistance → elevated insulin levels → additional storage of fat and increased appetite → more weight gain. Untreated, it just goes on and on until eventually your pancreas, the organ in your body responsible for producing insulin to keep your blood sugar in normal range, is unable to keep up with the demand. At this stage in the spectrum, blood sugars start to rise, first into the range of "prediabetes," and, ultimately, into overt diabetes. **So don't dismiss Syndrome W. It's not just a precursor to diabetes; it's your wake-up call!**

Two Variants on a Theme

Syndrome W has two file formats. Classic Syndrome W women are thin or normal weight most of their lives until they start to gain weight in their forties. (You can find many movie stars and former models who fit this mold.) A second group of women tell a different story. Women in this category describe a lifelong struggle with the scale. They typically report a best-case scenario of size 14 or even 16 (with great restraint and/or lots of exercise). At forty, their weight starts to spiral out of control as they add forty or fifty pounds, pushing them above the 40-plus size range. Unlike their lighter-weight sisters with classic Syndrome W, they find it increasingly difficult to stay with the stair-climber or aerobics classes, eventually abandoning all attempts to exercise. Decreased exercise and this increasingly sedentary lifestyle further aggravate overweight and obesity, eventually leading to serious secondary conditions, including:

- Respiratory (breathing) problems, even asthma
- Obstructive sleep apnea—breathing difficulties during sleep
- Joint (knee and hip) and back problems from excess weight with arthritis, ligament strains, and back injuries
- Blood sugar abnormalities
- Blood pressure elevations that require medication for control

If you're now topping the scales at 200 pounds or more, the Mogul Protocol will do more than reduce your dress size, it will add years to your life.

It really doesn't matter which weight group you start in. Either way, like so many of our highly successful patients, you'll be able to lose weight and gain health. But before you get started, you need to understand the Syndrome W cycle and a bit about its cause.

Location, Location, Location

Syndrome W is all about fat cells—when, where, and why you gain them. And it's also very much about what these fat cells *do* to increase the insulin resistance that drives Syndrome W onward and upward. You may even have read about this in cover stories in *Newsweek* magazine and the *New York Times* and features in *USA Today* or the health section of your local newspaper.

Fat cells are getting more and more of the blame, as the mysteries of our metabolism unfold. The problem is that all fat cells are not equal, and some (but not all) fat cells send out signals that start and sustain Syndrome W. To put it very simply, where you develop those first fat cells in your forties determines in large part whether you'll end up with Syndrome W. As you age, you gain weight for a number of reasons, including:

- Decreased physical activity (less time on the dance floor and sports field)
- Extra weight acquired in pregnancy in an era when doctors encouraged women to gain more weight than they needed for well-nourished babies
- Inadequate time to prepare and eat healthy food
- Overconsumption of fast food and supersize portions
- Genes that stored fat to enhance the likelihood of survival

Some women gain weight in the midsection of their bodies, adding new fat cells to their waists, inside their abdomens, and even in their liver. Unfortunately, fat cells in these locations have profoundly negative metabolic consequences, causing insulin resistance and increasing the risk of diabetes and heart disease.

Understanding Insulin Resistance

If you have insulin resistance, the insulin produced by your pancreas works *less efficiently* and *less effectively* than it should on certain "target" tissues (like your liver and your muscles). It encounters interference or "resistance" as it tries to do its major job—keeping your blood sugar in normal range by a diverse group of actions in various cells in your body—so that you don't develop diabetes (a disorder universally defined by blood sugar levels). However, your body has a great capacity to sense and compensate for most metabolic disturbances. So if you develop insulin resistance, your pancreas reads and responds to the danger down the road. It simply cranks up its output of insulin. This keeps your blood sugars at bay, but you pay. The cost is insulin elevation (also called hyperinsulinemia), especially when you eat sugar and carbohydrates.

Almost all women destined to develop diabetes go through the earlier Syndrome W stage—when they make a lot of insulin to keep their blood sugars in normal range. **The headlines following the first scientific presentation of Syndrome W capture this best: "'Syndrome' W Flags Insulin Resistance in Perimenopause" (page 1 of *Internal Medicine News*).**

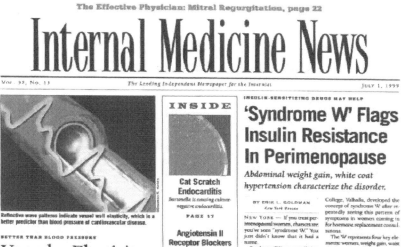

The Effective Physician: Mitral Regurgitation, page 22

Internal Medicine News

Vol. 32, No. 13   *The Leading Independent Newspaper for the Internist*   JULY 1, 1999

INSIDE

Reflective wave patterns indicate vessel wall elasticity, which is a better predictor than blood pressure of cardiovascular disease.

BETTER THAN BLOOD PRESSURE

Vascular Elasticity Predicts CVD Risk

BY ERIK L. GOLDMAN
New York Bureau

NEW YORK — Blood pressure measurements may soon take a backseat to direct vascular elas-... fatal cardiovascular events—in many cases of hypertension.

"Elevated blood pressure is not really the disease we're trying to treat. The disease is in the blood vessels. Blood pressure is a sur-...

Cat Scratch Endocarditis
Bartonella is causing culture negative endocarditis.
PAGE 17

Angiotensin II Receptor Blockers
"Sartans" work best for young hypertensive patients.
PAGE 20

INSULIN-SENSITIZING DRUGS MAY HELP

'Syndrome W' Flags Insulin Resistance In Perimenopause

Abdominal weight gain, white coat hypertension characterize the disorder.

BY ERIK L. GOLDMAN
New York Bureau

NEW YORK — If you treat perimenopausal women, chances are you've seen "syndrome W." You just didn't know that it had a name.

Syndrome W is a constellation of abdominal weight gain, appetite dysregulation, hyperinsulinemia, and intermittent hypertension in an otherwise healthy, active, euglycemic middle-aged patient, said Dr. Harriette Mogul who reported on 67 women with the syndrome at the annual meeting of the American Society of Endocrinology.

Dr. Mogul of the division of endocrinology, New York Medical College, Valhalla, developed the concept of syndrome W after repeatedly seeing this pattern of symptoms in women coming in for hormone replacement consultations.

The 'W' represents four key elements: women, weight gain, waist size increase, and white-coat hypertension. It is an early variant of syndrome X, a well-recognized disorder of insulin resistance.

She believes hyperinsulinemia, seen in 38 of the 67 women, is the underlying driver of this symptom aggregation and has found that drug and dietary interventions that decrease insulin levels will reduce both weight and blood pressure. These patients al-

See Perimenopause page 3

The hallmark of Syndrome W is hyperinsulinemia, elevated insulin levels above normal, expected values when you are fasting or during the performance of a glucose tolerance test (where blood tests are collected over a two-hour period after a sugar-loaded soda). Do not expect these abnormally high insulin levels to be found during any routine health evaluation. They'll remain undetected in almost any of you with Syndrome W because most physicians in the United States do not measure insulin levels, even in patients at high risk for insulin resistance or for type 2 diabetes.

Too Much of a Good Thing— Insulin, the Enemy Within

Unfortunately, as we are just beginning to understand, the extra insulin you make to maintain normal blood sugar has a life of its own. It acts in complex ways on other cells and tissues that are less insulin "resistant" than the cells that regulate blood sugar.

This produces a number of undesirable effects. High insulin levels can stimulate appetite and promote fat storage, both of which make it hard for you to lose weight. Thus, a vicious cycle is set in motion. Initial weight gain leads to:

- Increased insulin resistance
- That stimulates production of more insulin (hyperinsulinemia)
- That causes further fat storage *and* increased appetite
- That leads to more weight gain
- And on and on and on

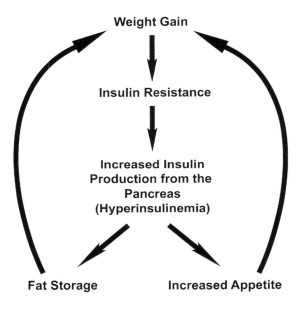

Reversing Course

We believe this is the mechanism of the upward weight spiral you've continued to experience—why you've become progressively more overweight each year despite all your efforts to diet and exercise and be more like your slimmer peers in our weight-obsessed society.

Metformin acts at all the points in this cycle. It decreases insulin resistance and reduces insulin levels, changing the direction of the spiral in the direction of the scale. It is truly a miracle medication, the missing link that unlocks the weight-gain puzzle of Syndrome W and makes all the difference by enhancing all those weight-loss strategies you've tried that didn't work before.

Metformin and the dietary program that make up the Mogul Protocol represent a unique approach to midlife weight gain with a

different goal—targeting and treating the underlying insulin resistance and hyperinsulinemia that cause Syndrome W. It's more like treating a cold, rather than treating cold symptoms. This combo regimen contrasts with other diet- and exercise-based weight-loss plans with notably low long-term success rates because it was specifically designed to fix the defects responsible for the disorder.

Now, for the first time ever, you can mend your metabolism with a safe and inexpensive medication and an easy-to-follow, healthy, enjoyable, nondeprivation diet—a combination that gives you lots of additional benefits because metformin also:

- Prevents progression of hyperinsulinemia to diabetes.
- Lowers your blood pressure.
- Improves the balance of good and bad cholesterol and triglycerides (other fats) in the bloodstream.
- Reduces the risk of cardiovascular disease.

Early identification and treatment of Syndrome W are critical to your weight *and* your health. Now that you understand the cause and implications of Syndrome W, you can see how metformin and the Carb-Modified Diet can offer new hope in halting your progressive weight spiral.

You will find nothing more motivating than seeing that first ten-pound loss after metformin lowers your insulin levels and controls your food cravings. Now you can finally eliminate the frustration and hopelessness of progressive midlife weight gain, and this time it can be forever.

Part II

your answer:
The Mogul Protocol

When you sign on to the Mogul Protocol, you'll be using a two-pronged program designed to work in tandem to target and treat the cause of weight gain in Syndrome W women as well as other overweight insulin-resistant Americans. You follow an eating plan called the Carb-Modified Diet, and you take the medication metformin, which is a well-known, highly effective drug that's been used worldwide to treat millions of people with diabetes for many years. In part II, you will read about the widely cited study that first suggested metformin could be used as a primary treatment of obesity, and you'll read stories of women with Syndrome W who "led the way" in motivating me to add metformin as they gained weight despite low-calorie diet and exercise regimens that exceeded public health guidelines for weight reduction. And you'll get the lowdown on metformin and Syndrome X (the very serious metabolic disorder that evolves when women fail to get Syndrome W diagnosed and treated early).

Chapter 8

CONNECTING THE DOTS

Making Sense of What You Thought Was Nonsensical

IF YOU HAVE SYNDROME W, you're probably astonished that a diagnosis *with a solution* could be close at hand. So you can imagine my surprise when we first looked at data from our patients and discovered the patterns that paved the way to finding and defining Syndrome W.

Like so many discoveries in science, finding Syndrome W was somewhat serendipitous. I had two things going for me: my feminist perspective and the power of the (female) press—a page-one feature in the *New York Times*. The writer, Kate Lombardi, described our menopausal health program, which was designed to evaluate risk factors and individualize hormone replacement and other lifestyle interventions in midlife women. This article touched a chord and brought a deluge—hundreds of health-conscious perimenopausal women seeking a "health risk appraisal" and advice on estrogen use. A predominantly healthy contingent, these females in their forties and fifties made an ideal group for gathering information about menopause in the contemporary United States. Characteristics that most of them shared were the following:

- They were bright and well informed about health issues.
- They routinely exercised and dieted.
- They didn't complain of hot flashes.
- They *did* complain of weight gain.

Fortuitously, about this same time, many people nationwide were scrutinizing some interesting new data from the important Nurses' Health Study at Harvard. Just released, the Nurses' Health Study showed that midlife weight gain in women didn't appear as benign as physicians had always believed. Reports in the prestigious *Journal of the American Medical Association* and *The New England Journal of Medicine* maintained that even modest weight gain—as little as twenty additional pounds in women in their forties and fifties—could dramatically increase their rates of diabetes, heart disease, and death from all causes.

In response to this riveting information, my clinic instituted three key moves:

1. We added a simple question to our intake questionnaire: "Have you gained twenty pounds since you were in your twenties?"
2. We recommended a two-hour glucose tolerance test for all nondiabetic women who responded yes. (This would help us evaluate the risk of diabetes and heart disease—important factors in determining whether estrogen use was appropriate.)
3. We measured insulin levels during the test. (Insulin elevations in response to sugar load are the earliest clinically detectable signs of impending type 2 diabetes.)

Who Knew?

Our findings were astonishing and entirely unexpected. More than one-third (105 of 277) of our healthy, health-conscious, nondiabetic patients had very abnormal insulin curves. What was most surprising was that in the group of women who were overweight to mildly obese (BMIs of 25 to 32 kg/m^2), very few had any blood sugar abnormality on the glucose tolerance tests. In fact, more than 90 percent of them had completely textbook-normal glucose tolerance curves.

So we didn't find the diabetes we were looking for. Instead, what surfaced was an epidemic of hyperinsulinemia in a large group of "healthy" women who had gained more than twenty pounds since their twenties.

These results were very exciting for several reasons. We could now identify which overweight women most urgently needed to lose weight. It also allowed us to separate our overweight patients into two groups:

- Women with "cosmetic" obesity who had normal insulin levels
- Women with Syndrome W whose weight reduction was critical to preserve quality and quantity of life

Something Old Is New Again

Fortunately, I already had in hand what I considered perfect ammo for addressing the weight problem of Syndrome W—a diet tailor-made for women with hyperinsulinemia. Devised twenty years earlier, the Carb-Modified Diet featured the following elements:

- Lots of vegetables and low-fat proteins
- Limited starches and fats
- Strict curtailment of sugar

Designed to lower insulin levels, this eating plan capitalized on the benefits of low-glycemic-index (high-fiber) diets. It also fit nicely with new dietary recommendations and data lauding the health benefits of a Mediterranean-type diet to prevent heart disease and cancer. So all we needed was a copy machine and just a bit of counseling to launch the Carb-Modified Diet in our Syndrome W women. Carbohydrate cravings decreased, and the weight gain slowed down in most of the women.

But something was still missing. Most of the women were still unable to lose weight. Many women insisted that no matter how strictly they followed the diet, their food cravings never completely subsided, and when I looked at the food journals I'd advised the women to keep, I saw a disconnect between calories in and pounds off. **It became increasingly clear that something was still missing for a successful Syndrome W solution.**

Chapter 9

CREATING THE MOGUL PROTOCOL

Women Led the Way

MY PATIENTS TAUGHT ME WHAT WORKED and what didn't for
women with midlife weight gain and Syndrome W. Their disappoint-
ment over continued weight gain, even after following the Carb-
Modified Diet, was ultimately responsible for the creation of the
Mogul Protocol. It turned out to be the right plan for the right time.

The Pain of Gain

Bobby is a perfect example. Curious about estrogen options, she first came
to our menopausal health program in 1995. Formerly normal-weight,
Bobby had become alarmed when she experienced a dramatic forty-
pound weight gain in her forties. She went from size 12 to 20-plus. When I
first met her, she was classic Syndrome W and very disturbed about being
overweight. At the outset, her main complaints were typical menopausal
symptoms: hot flashes, night sweats, and disturbed sleep patterns.

Though significantly overweight, Bobby was a strikingly beautiful woman with a poised, quiet manner that seemed at odds with her
high-level position as an administrator of a busy clinical program at our
hospital. A fanciful and careful wardrobe helped to hide the 24 percent
weight increase of the past five years. Blood tests, used to decide whether
estrogen replacement was right for her, revealed that Bobby had:

- A slightly elevated (though normal) fasting blood sugar.
- High cholesterol and triglycerides.

- Lower HDL (good) cholesterol than desirable for a midforties female.

And the results of a glucose tolerance test (to get a better measure of her risk for type 2 diabetes) showed impaired glucose tolerance (IGT), an early variant of type 2 diabetes (long considered a prediabetic condition).

Using clinical guidelines of the time, I suggested a strict weight-loss program. I gave her a copy of the Carb-Modified Diet, nutritional/behavioral counseling, and an estrogen patch for the menopausal symptoms and asked her to return for periodic follow-up visits so that we could check on her diet progress and her estrogen management.

Over the next two years, I shared Bobby's bewilderment as I watched her tack on an additional twenty-five pounds despite her resolve to lose weight, lower her cholesterol and triglycerides, and prevent development of diabetes. The estrogen patch made her feel better, and she was doing more exercise than I had recommended. She faithfully took low-calorie lunches to work. But her weight continued to climb. Thyroid tests, checked repeatedly, failed to provide an explanation for pounds that seemed out of proportion to her dietary intake. And the sincerity of her strong desire to lose weight stood in stark contrast to her progressive gain.

Nothing worked, neither intensive individual nutritional and behavioral strategies nor her participation in Weight Watchers. Finally, with her blood sugars soaring toward diabetic range, Bobby had full-fledged metabolic syndrome (also called Syndrome X, described in chapter 13). I was concerned that we were running out of time for intervention, so I decided to try one more trick. I suggested we add a diabetes medication called metformin to the mix. After two years of determined but unsuccessful dieting, Bobby agreed that it was time for an alternate approach.

We started with one tablet a day (about a quarter of the dose to control diabetes), which we increased gradually in order to avoid stomach upsets associated with metformin. This type of dosing made it easy to monitor any effects of metformin on kidney and liver function, appetite, and food cravings at regular treatment intervals.

By the time she took her third tablet, Bobby reported a profound reduction in appetite. With the fourth tablet, she was amazed that she no longer felt hungry all the time, and her food cravings practically disappeared. As I now tell all new patients, it's not that you don't have to "diet" or reduce caloric intake to lose weight with the Mogul Protocol—it's just that the metformin and the elimination of food cravings make it a lot easier to stay on a diet and lose weight.

You may even have seen Bobby's story on "Doctor's Diary" on the Health Network in a ten-episode series that chronicled physicians and their patients from our Westchester Medical Center in New York. Bobby was delighted to appear in a patient vignette; she didn't seem to mind one bit that the camera crew was posting her weight chart, recounting for viewers worldwide the details of her forty-pound weight loss and her exact weight at that time.

In the five years since then, Bobby has lost twenty more pounds and wears a size 14. She still follows the Carb-Modified Diet. Without intending to, she accidentally became the poster child for the Mogul Protocol. Of course, Bobby's success inspired me to add metformin to the dietary regimen of other nondiabetic women with hyperinsulinemia who clearly needed more than just diet.

Midlife Malaise

Ally was another early patient who was a more classic Syndrome W. At age forty-eight, she weighed in at 155 on her first visit to our menopausal health program. Believe me, she was not a happy woman!

Two issues prompted her visit. A six-month trial of a commonly prescribed pill for menopause had done nothing for troublesome hot flashes, and she had gained ten pounds in the prior year despite an active lifestyle (regular aerobics classes and tennis). Plus, she insisted her diet was healthy and basically unchanged from what she had eaten most of her adult life, when she had always maintained a weight of 120.

What most distressed Ally was that she was continuing to outgrow her clothes every six months. She had gone from size 6 to "almost" 16. "I can't even find clothes that fit in the stores in town," she told us. She also reported being "a little hungrier than in the past." Her major concern, though, was that she had run out of ideas for losing weight.

Oddly enough, Ally didn't look very overweight. In fact, at five feet five, she had a body mass index (BMI) of 25.8, only slightly above normal. Her arms and legs were slim and muscled, but all of her weight was concentrated at her thirty-four-inch waist.

Ally's blood pressure of 140/82 was hardly a cause for alarm, but it was many points higher than the 90/70 low blood pressure recordings of her youth (even during pregnancy).

I suggested that we do a glucose tolerance test to see whether she had the insulin abnormality that signals Syndrome W. It showed that

Ally had a textbook-perfect glucose curve: a fasting blood sugar of 80, a half-hour peak of 120, and a two-hour value of 80. But she also had high insulin levels in response to this glucose "challenge." At all time periods, her insulin levels were clearly abnormal, with a one-hour peak of 100 and a total value above 140.

Like many of my patients, Ally had to fight back tears when I told her that the test results revealed the cause for her twenty-five-pound weight accumulation—hyperinsulinemia.

I switched Ally's hormone regimen to an estrogen patch (because it causes less weight gain than oral estrogen) and micronized proges-terone, which decreases two-hour insulin. I also suggested that she continue to attend weekly Weight Watchers meetings with her hus-band but substitute our Carb-Modified Diet to reduce her insulin levels. I asked her to come back to see us in six months to evaluate her progress on all fronts.

I ran into Ally at a charity dinner a few months later, and she told me that she felt much better but still had to struggle to fit into her clothes. Her trim husband reported that he had lost twenty pounds on the Carb-Modified Diet even though Ally, who was much stricter and ate far less, wasn't losing any weight.

At her six-month visit, Ally had gained five more pounds, despite all attempts to diet and daily intense exercise. I agreed that we were going "nowhere but up." So I explained to Ally that I'd started to use a drug called metformin to treat women who had all the following char-acteristics:

- Evidence of insulin resistance on their glucose tolerance tests
- Other signs of Syndrome W: blood pressure increases or waistlines in an unhealthy range (larger than thirty-five inches, as defined by National Institutes of Health guidelines)
- Failure to lose weight after six months of structured or medically supervised diets

I explained that metformin, which had been widely used to treat diabetes in Europe and had just gotten approval in the United States, was the first drug to treat insulin resistance and was known to lower the insulin levels that I thought were the culprit and cause of Syndrome W. I emphasized that we would be using metformin "off label" as an anti-obesity drug and reviewed its potential side effects and risks. I added two 500 mg tablets to Ally's Carb-Modified Diet, and I asked her to check her blood chemistries and her fasting insulin in four weeks, prior to a return visit a month later. The Mogul Protocol was launched!

Five weeks later Ally was all smiles as she walked into my examining room. She stuck her thumb into her waistband and told me that for the first time in months, her size 14 pants were a lot looser at the waist. She reported that she had a detectable change in appetite and was definitely eating less overall. I congratulated her on a six-pound weight loss and noted a dip in her blood pressure to 120/78. I increased her metformin to three tablets a day to further normalize her fasting insulin, which had declined by 25 percent but was still elevated. I asked her to return in three months.

I needed to see Ally only three more times that year. At her one-year follow-up, her weight was down to 126 pounds and she was able to wear "all those great outfits stored at the back of the closet." Her fasting insulin had declined 42 percent from baseline and was well into the normal range; her blood pressure was 110/74. I gave her a six-month prescription for metformin (three times a day) and renewed her hormone replacement.

I no longer see Ally as a patient because her primary care physician has assumed responsibility for what is truly just "health maintenance." He now prescribes the medications she started at our menopausal health program. However, I run into her every year or so at local charity events. She always pushes her way through the crowd, bypassing en route all those hors d'oeuvres that she learned to avoid, eager to show me that she remains a model patient in all respects—slimmer, trimmer, and very happy about it all.

So Many Symptoms, So Little Time

These two success stories show how easy it is to overlook Syndrome W early in the weight spiral, when doctors may not be impressed with your symptoms. This means *you* may need to take the initiative to find your own answers, especially if you're not very overweight and look healthy in the eyes of physicians long accustomed to caring for more obese women with *overt* signs of diabetes and heart disease.

Your complaints of expanding girth and those few extra digits in your blood pressure can easily fall on deaf ears. With a 12-ish figure and a weight in the low 150s, you're not very overweight by current U.S.

standards. You may not even look fat unless your doctor looks carefully and finds those pinchable inches around your midsection that obliterate your waistline or, better yet, uses a tape measure to record your exact waist circumference.

The Mogul Protocol—metformin and the Carb-Modified Diet—can reverse Syndrome W as dramatically as it appears, but you have to find the syndrome before you can fix it. Then you, too, can join the ranks of women like Ally, who's still wearing size-10 pants after more than ten years on our regimen. You really can reverse midlife weight gain and become healthier and happier as you take control.

Chapter 10

DEFINING SYNDROME W AND GOING PUBLIC

Sharing Information with Those Who Need It

YOU MAY LIKE THE CAMARADERIE of reading about women you can relate to, but you probably want to see some data. My well-informed patients frequently ask for "the latest findings from research." So let's look at the scoreboard. As an epidemiologist, I'll have to say that I was a bit hesitant to report the results of a "case series" before we had a chance to conduct a clinical trial—one of those randomized studies that are critical to testing new therapies.

However, by 2001, the obesity epidemic was reaching new proportions. The U.S. population was growing fatter, as shown by each national survey. Medication was increasingly recommended as an adjunct to diet and exercise regimens; but physicians had few effective and acceptable therapies to advocate even though they were becoming extremely worried about the dramatic rise in obesity and diabetes in Americans of all ages, including children.

Motivated by the high rate of success and the ease of using the Mogul Protocol, I felt that it was important to go public and release our preliminary findings to the attention and scrutiny of the scientific and medical communities.

Summarizing Success

Data from patients who had used the Mogul Protocol exceeded all expectations, including the following:

- Weight loss in 90 percent of twenty-eight midlife nondiabetic women (with an average BMI of 36 kg/m²) two to three times greater than typically reported in other studies, in which patients were seen more often and followed for shorter periods
- A striking reduction in food cravings reported in all of the women
- No significant side effects to the medication
- Marked improvements in fasting insulin levels, blood pressure, HDL (good) cholesterol, and triglycerides, typically in the normal range

These improvements in classic risk factors for heart disease were much higher than expected, considering the modest changes in weight. However, the most important finding by far was our data from the six-month follow-up visit after the women had completed the formal one-year treatment program. Almost all (eight of nine) women who continued metformin didn't regain any weight, whereas most (five of six) women who stopped the medication (and continued the diet alone) regained the weight they had lost.

Moving Out with Metformin

Clearly, metformin made all the difference in the program.

Metformin, used widely in Europe, first became available in the United States in 1995 (see chapter 12 for additional details). A unique diabetes drug, metformin is what's termed an "insulin sensitizer." It works by a different mechanism than do other oral diabetes medications. Metformin doesn't lower blood sugar by stimulating the pancreas to produce more insulin. Metformin decreases insulin resistance, the key defect in diabetes, mainly by decreasing the amount of sugar produced by the liver when we sleep. So the net result of metformin differs from the effects of other diabetes drugs; it lowers (rather than increases) insulin levels.

Studies have demonstrated other benefits of metformin:

- It improves the cardiovascular risk profile in diabetics.
- It prevents the progression to diabetes in prediabetics.
- It reduces appetite in diabetics and nondiabetics.

Nonetheless, like all medications, metformin had side effects, including a rare but potentially serious side effect called "lactic acidosis." So I was initially reluctant to use it "off label," as a primary treatment for obesity even in women with documented insulin abnormalities.

Ultimately, my patients made the choice. Once we identified Syndrome W, I presented two options: a three- to six-month trial of the Carb-Modified Diet with or without the addition of metformin. I explained that we would be using the medication "off label," reviewed its known risks and benefits, and gave our patients a written sheet detailing directions for starting and stopping metformin (reproduced in chapter 12).

We presented our "Preliminary Findings from a Case Series" in a peer-reviewed journal (Mogul et al. 2001) after we collected data on the first twenty-eight women who started treatment and "returned for at least one follow-up visit."

When our results were released, the scientific community responded positively to our preliminary study—the first ever to suggest that metformin in combination with our Carb-Modified Diet could be used as a primary obesity treatment. Just days after the study's publication, it was picked up by Reuters and *Medscape's Diabetes and Endocrinology* weekly online coverage of medical highlights (November 2001). Articles in the *New York Times* and health columns in the *Wall Street Journal* still refer to our study, which remains the first report in the medical literature of metformin as a primary obesity treatment.

Since that publication just a few years ago, hundreds of women, men, and children have lost weight and kept it off when treated by physicians using the Mogul Protocol.

So it's time to get ready—now it's your turn.

Chapter 11

MOVING BEYOND CLASSIC SYNDROME W WITH OTHER CHRONICLES

Beyond the Healthy White Women from Our First Report

MY VISION OF SYNDROME W changed after looking at the prevalence of Syndrome W in our community-based Weight Management Clinic at Westchester Medical Center (WMC). Syndrome W was far more widespread and untreated than even I had imagined. In our first report, where the majority (97.5 percent) of the women were white, Syndrome W was diagnosed in approximately one out of six women, whereas when we looked at our WMC population, we found that it occurred in about nine of ten nondiabetic women ages thirty to sixty-five, including 86 percent of nonwhite women and 100 percent of the small number of Latinas we tested. Indeed, Syndrome W was epidemic among overweight and obese Westchesterites, affecting adults and adolescents of all ethnicities, socioeconomic groups, and education levels. This included hospital staff administrators, doctors, nurses, and women from as far away as India and Africa.

The WMC experience opened my eyes and those of other attending physicians and physicians-in-training who staffed the clinic, as we saw the alarming frequency of insulin abnormalities in adults and adolescents with no sign whatsoever of diabetes on routine blood sugar tests. The high rates of Syndrome W in African American and Hispanic American women—two- to threefold higher than in our original group of white women—indicated that Syndrome W was both widespread and underrecognized. These observations, along with the high success rate of our early patients, served as impetus to spread the word about Syndrome W. The women we saw at WMC were the driving forces for this book.

The Hispanic Connection

Liz and Luisa are two women with unusual Syndrome W stories. Ten years and more than twenty pounds apart, they are both examples of the epidemic of Syndrome W among Hispanic American women in my practice and in their counterparts in Puerto Rico and Peru.

When Liz was in her early thirties, she came in expressing concern over unusual fatigue, a "possible thyroid abnormality," and "problems losing weight." She had a family history of thyroid disease (all the women in her family) and wondered whether she needed thyroid medication. She told me that she worked out regularly and didn't eat as much as most people she knew.

Her exam revealed a nodular thyroid and a thirty-two-inch waist, a little large for her size-10 frame. I ordered thyroid tests, including antibodies that can indicate a chronic thyroid problem. And because of her "weight problem" and the fact that her good cholesterol (HDL) was significantly lower than I expected in a thirty-something exercising woman, I asked her whether she wanted to have a glucose tolerance and insulin test.

As expected, Liz had thyroiditis (a common condition in women), with mildly decreased levels of thyroid hormone. To my surprise, however, she also had high insulin levels (with a totally normal glucose tolerance test).

I gave Liz the Carb-Modified Diet, urged her to step up her exercise a bit, and added the thyroid medication that I hoped might facilitate weight loss. Liz followed all my instructions, lost "those ten extra pounds," and regained her size-8 to -10 waistline. Her fasting insulin, which was monitored annually along with her thyroid, remained normal after her first visit.

For seven years, I saw Liz annually, and on each visit, I praised her dedication to lifestyle change. Then, near her fortieth birthday, Liz returned for her yearly checkup, complaining of hot flashes of early menopause. She was also worried about the ten pounds she'd gained in the past year, but she insisted that she had changed nothing in her diet or exercise patterns.

Sure enough, Liz's fasting insulin had crept up more than 25 percent since her prior visit, and her repeat glucose tolerance and insulin response curves were now abnormal. I suggested metformin, and she agreed that this was probably the best way to halt her progressive weight gain since she was already dieting.

Liz did well with the addition of metformin. When she returned three months after starting medication, we discussed the incidence of Syndrome W in Hispanic women, and I asked her to estimate the percentage of nondiabetic Hispanic women with hyperinsulinemia whom we had found in our community clinic. She said "100 percent" with certainty, and she was right. She added that she had just returned from Puerto Rico, where all the women in their thirties had expanding waistlines and narrow hips and spoke of their frustrating, unsuccessful attempts to diet and exercise.

Luisa, a computer analyst who had climbed the ranks from clerk to executive VP at a local corporation, was another example. She'd been overweight most of her life but had managed to stay between size 14 and 16 by doing lots of exercise and eating properly. Luisa was tall and muscular, but she topped the scale at close to two hundred pounds at her first visit. She had seen one of our patients lose weight in the past year and wondered whether she might also have "that Syndrome W thing." In fact, she already had copies of our diet, which she was attempting to follow, but wanted "something else" to curb her "constant weight gain and out-of-control, too-healthy appetite."

When Luisa's insulin levels came back elevated, she, like so many other patients, choked back tears. After adding metformin, Luisa lost thirty pounds the first year, and she has never gone back. A new body and increased self-esteem led her to make some long-overdue changes in her personal life (getting rid of a ne'er-do-well boyfriend). An ideal patient, Luisa is a terrific example of the American dream. I smile when she walks into my exam room each year when I see her long-term weight maintenance, and I share her joy in the success she has had on all fronts.

If you are Hispanic or Mexican American or from any country in South or Central America or a neighboring island, and you have the symptoms of Syndrome W—or if you have a history of polycystic ovarian syndrome (PCOS), *or* if you had a baby that weighed more than nine pounds at birth, *or* if you had a "slightly abnormal glucose tolerance test during pregnancy," you are at high risk for Syndrome W *even if your blood sugar is now completely normal*. Ask your doctor to order a glucose tolerance test—this time, **with insulin levels.**

Shirley's Story: Syndrome W in African Americans

I first met Shirley, an African American nurse, during a media interview after she had lost 171 pounds at our hospital-based weight management program. I had heard all about her phenomenal progress under the care of one of our program's primary care physicians and had followed her story as her weight declined in the eighteen months since she first came "up to Westchester" from her neighborhood health center.

I knew that Shirley was an excellent example of how well our methods work—and how the program stands tall as a viable alternative to the use of bariatric surgery in the treatment of what I prefer to call "extreme" obesity. But I wasn't prepared for the intense emotional impact of this truly special woman. Here is her story as she told it to the readers of the *Journal News*.

Like many overweight or obese African American women I see, Shirley didn't have the blood sugar abnormalities that we have been taught to expect in a population at high risk for diabetes. She is truly proof positive that, like women of other ethnicities, black women can have insulin abnormalities without any evidence of blood sugar disturbances.

Compared with the other Syndrome W women, many of the African American women we see have a different Syndrome W profile. Typically, they have high blood pressure, but they also have better HDL (good) cholesterol levels, and they lack the characteristic waist gain and the pregnant appearance seen in most other women with Syndrome W. If you are African American and have gained twenty pounds or more since your twenties, understand that it may be even harder for you (or your doctors) to detect and correct Syndrome W.

Diabetes pills spur weight loss

Metformin, diet low in carbs help woman take off 160 pounds

Melissa Klein
The Journal News

In an era when gastric surgery has helped thousands of obese people peel off pounds, Shirley Williams has instead dieted her way down the scale to a weight she hasn't seen in so many years, she can't remember when.

What finally helped the 58-year-old Mount Vernon resident lose 160 pounds was a low-carbohydrate eating plan, a medication commonly given to diabetics and her own perseverance to finally take off the weight.

"I just got to the point in my mind where I said I can't take it anymore," Williams said.

Williams, who at 5 feet 2 inches tall had reached 460 pounds, was found to have what has been called "Syndrome W," weight gain accompanied by an abnormally high level of insulin.

The syndrome was first identified about eight years ago by Dr. Harriette Mogul, an endocrinologist and director of the Weight Management Program at Westchester Medical Center in Valhalla, after the hospital opened a menopause center.

"We ended up with hundreds and hundreds of women who wanted appointments," Mogul said. "Their complaints really were not hot flashes."

Instead, the women, most of whom had been thin, complained of weight gain that started after their 40th birthdays, particularly around their waists, that they just couldn't lose. They also said they had an increase in appetite and food cravings.

Mogul found that the women had normal blood-sugar levels, meaning they were not diabetic, but had high levels of insulin, a problem known as insulin resistance.

Please see DIABETES, 2B

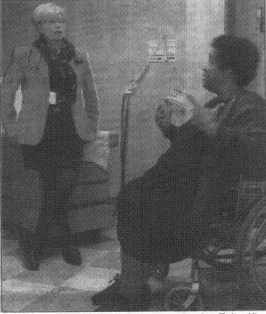

Stuart Bayer/The Journal News
Endocrinologist Dr. Harriette Mogul, left, talks with Shirley Williams of Mount Vernon at the Westchester Medical Center in Valhalla. Williams lost 160 pounds through a weight program created by Mogul.

Atkins stands by protein-diet plan

Melissa Klein
The Journal News

VALHALLA — Diet doctor Robert Atkins asked for a show of hands among the medical students, residents and doctors gathered yesterday in a lecture hall at New York Medical College.

"How many people heard that our diet is dangerous?" he asked.

At least half the hands inside the packed auditorium went up.

"Whoever didn't raise your hand must have a hearing difficulty," Atkins joked.

Atkins was ridiculed by the medical establishment when he published his diet 30 years ago. His book told people that carbohydrates were the cause of their weight gain and advocated an eating plan that relied on protein, including such high-fat foods as steak and butter. The Atkins plan still has detractors, but an increasing number of experts are agreeing with the notion that the nation's obesity epidemic has

Please see DIET, 2B

"I just got to the point in my mind where I said I can't take it anymore."
Shirley Williams

Women Tipping the Scales at Two Hundred Plus

Everything we've covered so far pertains to classic Syndrome W women—ones who were basically thin or normal-weight adults before their upward weight spirals. They generally walk into our office with a body mass index (BMI) in the overweight-to-obese category (25–35 kg/m²).

But women who weigh in at two hundred pounds plus or have a BMI greater than 35 kg/m² may be wondering where they fit in. If you fit in this higher-weight range, you probably are insulin resistant, and you may even have some subtle or not-so-subtle abnormalities in your glucose tolerance tests as well. If you weigh two hundred or more and you can't seem to lose weight even though your blood sugar level is normal range, your score on the Syndrome W scale is superfluous. No doubt about it, you need to talk to your doctor about additional tests and treatment ASAP.

Debby was a patient of ours from this two hundred–plus group, and she had a happy outcome to what started out as a grim weight story. Debby, a lawyer who had three children, came to our practice for help losing weight after she saw one of her coworkers lose thirty pounds and keep it off with our treatment regimen. Debby wasn't sure she could be helped because she had already tried "every diet there was." She (like many of my patients of her generation and genealogy who grew up on the West Side of Manhattan) had a slim mother who dragged her to her first diet doctor when Debby was a slightly overweight preteen ("only a size 14 at the time").

Debby had maintained her weight in college and law school by "starving and smoking" and had lost and gained hundreds of pounds in a lifetime of diets and weight cycling. She tried liquid diets, Duke, and fen-phen and was even considering gastric bypass surgery. Her primary care doctor was concerned about new blood pressure elevations and suggested that it was time for her "to get serious about losing weight." Although Debby was exercising an hour a day and seeing a nutritionist, nothing was working.

Like many other high-achieving women with undetected hyperinsulinemia, Debby blushed and fought back tears when I explained her test results. (I've learned to keep tissues on my desk.) Her words echoed those of so many other women with PhDs, MBAs, LLBs, and MDs who are supersuccessful and good at controlling all aspects of their lives except weight. They all said, "I just knew all along something had to be wrong!"—and they were right.

After one year of taking metformin and following the Carb-Modified Diet, Debby lost more than 15 percent of her body weight. Now, after three years of follow-up, like many other "near-diabetic" women in this weight range whom I see twice a year, she has lost more than sixty pounds (25 percent of her initial weight). My long-term fifty-plus-pound winners all agree that such progress had previously been out of the question unless they restricted their eating almost to the point of starvation.

High-Risk Syndrome W

So there's no question that Syndrome W is a ubiquitous perimenopausal phenomenon that can be seen not just in the predominantly (97.5 percent) white women from our first report but in women of all ethnicities. As you can imagine, although the identification of the syndrome is important for all women, the need to find and fix it is critical in African American, Hispanic, and very overweight women, all of whom have a higher than average risk of developing diabetes down the road.

Starting the Mogul Protocol in high-risk Syndrome W women addresses far more than weight. Metformin targets and treats their underlying insulin resistance, prevents the progression to diabetes, and decreases many of the related manifestations of Syndrome X described in chapter 13.

If you have Syndrome W and/or documented insulin abnormalities after your glucose tolerance test and are African American, Hispanic, or very overweight, it is imperative that you start to reverse the syndrome as soon as you can. Like so many nonclassic Syndrome W women, you can lose weight and gain health with the Mogul Protocol.

Listen Up

By now you can see that the message is clear: progressive weight gain—the extra twenty to fifty pounds most women gain when a switch goes off at forty—is *not* an inevitable consequence of aging, especially if you used to be a thin to normal-weight woman and if you eat well and/or exercise.

Look at Syndrome W as a detectable and correctable metabolic defect. As headlined, Syndrome W flags insulin resistance in perimenopause at a stage when it is still reversible. Discovering that you have Syndrome W gives you an explanation and an intervention that will help you get a handle on your weight for life.

About 90 percent of women (with BMIs in the 25–35 kg/m² range who return for two or more follow-up visits) lose an average of 13 to 15 percent of their initial weight, typically twenty-five to forty pounds, in one year. Some have lost more than one hundred pounds. This includes pre- and postmenopausal women, men and adolescents, and even extremely obese patients with life-threatening obesity, like the patients I first met in medical school almost forty years ago who motivated my quest for answers. **Most importantly, in virtually all our patients who have lost weight and whom we follow annually (some up to ten years now), the weight loss has been permanent.**

Chapter 12

THE LOWDOWN ON METFORMIN

Understanding Metformin Is Essential to Your Health

Get Your Doctor on Board and Online

IF YOUR DOCTOR hasn't heard about the Mogul Protocol or the use of metformin to treat obesity in people with insulin resistance, encourage him to access our publications on websites like PubMed or Medline. Selected publications can also be downloaded with a simple click on our website, www.SyndromeW.com, or retrieved on Google. Most physicians are happy to have new tools to treat obesity, and I frequently get requests for copies of our protocol and diet materials from doctors as far away as Argentina and Russia. I'm sure your doctor will be pleased to learn that details of our soon-to-be-completed multicenter randomized clinical trial, EMPOWIR: Enhance the Metabolic Profile of Women with Insulin Resistance, are available at ClinicalTrials. gov, registration number NCT00618072. EMPOWIR is based on all the principles in these chapters and represents the first test of our methods in this era of evidence-based medicine.

Why Metformin?

Metformin is FDA approved as the number one oral drug for mono-therapy (single medication) diabetes treatment in the United States and is widely advocated as "first line therapy" by official diabetes organizations worldwide. Large clinical studies have verified metformin's effectiveness and safety based on use in millions of diverse diabetics. In addition to its primary action in improving blood sugar control, metformin also significantly lowered the risk of cardiovascular disease and improved life expectancy in diabetic populations.

Metformin delayed the onset of diabetes in high-risk individuals evaluated in a large diabetes prevention trial. The American Diabetes Association currently recommends metformin treatment for patients with documented "prediabetes" (defined by a fasting blood sugar greater than 100 mg/dL in combination with a two-hour blood sugar greater than 140 mg/dL) who fail to respond to a six-month program of diet and exercise.

The metabolic effects of metformin in nondiabetics were recently evaluated in what we call a meta-analysis, a study in which data from numerous studies are pooled together to produce a single summary measure. **The analysis looked at all placebo-controlled randomized clinical trials of metformin in nondiabetics conducted in the past forty years** (1966 to 2006), yielding summary data from a total of 4,570 study participants followed for a total of 8,267 patient-years. The authors found metformin significantly reduced body weight; lowered the risk of diabetes; and improved cardiovascular risk factors. Body mass index decreased by 5 percent, fasting insulin decreased by 14.4 percent, and HOMA, a well-known, commonly used measure of insulin resistance, decreased by 22.6 percent! Progression to diabetes was reduced by 40 percent. They concluded that metformin may have important benefits for high-risk women and men with insulin resistance.

Mechanisms for That Metabolic Makeover

Metformin acts in multiple ways to decrease insulin resistance, lower insulin levels, and reduce appetite. One of a new category of drugs termed "insulin sensitizers," metformin makes the insulin produced by your body work more efficiently and more effectively to maintain normal blood sugars throughout the day. Metformin doesn't increase the amount of insulin produced by your pancreas, like earlier traditional diabetes drugs (called "oral hypoglycemic agents"). **Metformin reduces insulin resistance—the major defect in people with type 2 diabetes.** It acts predominantly at the liver to reduce the amount of sugar that circulates in the bloodstream before eating. In contrast to the first generation of diabetes drugs, metformin decreases the body's production (or over-production) of insulin, ultimately lowering your insulin levels.

We also know that metformin reduces the free fatty acids that are associated with diabetes' serious consequences (heart disease and other large blood vessel disorders).

In the past decade, we've learned a lot more about where metformin acts and what it does in the liver, the brain, and the gut. One of the newly described mechanisms relates to the effect of metformin on a major appetite-regulating protein called ghrelin. (See also chapter 19.) This "hunger hormone" rises after each meal and falls when we eat. Studies show that fasting levels of ghrelin are high in obese people and are lowered via bariatric surgery, which partly explains why operations that reduce stomach size cause weight loss. A recent study showed that metformin significantly reduced ghrelin levels in overweight subjects.

This fits well with previous studies that show metformin decreases appetite and reduces food intake in both diabetics and nondiabetics and it's great news for your weight-loss regimen. We know we've reached the right dose when our patients tell us they're "no longer starving all the time!" The welcomed side effect of decreased hunger/cravings is very direct and rapid. Conversely, food cravings return rapidly when metformin is stopped.

Metformin is not a "magic bullet" for weight loss, but added to the Carb-Modified Diet, it *is* the missing link for midlife women or men, adolescents, and elders with insulin resistance and elevated insulin levels.

Metformin Modes and Methods

Metformin is available in several forms:

- Regular metformin—a generic, immediate-release form available in 500 mg doses
- Metformin XR—a generic form of extended-release metformin (previously marketed as Glucophage, manufactured by Bristol-Myers Squibb)—available in doses of 500 mg, 850 mg, and 1000 mg
- Fortamet and Glumetza—two extended-release formulations that are released slowly throughout the stomach and upper gastrointestinal track and typically cause fewer gastrointestinal

side effects. They are more expensive than generic extended-release forms and almost always require higher copayments. Of particular note is the fact that these formulations do not contain gluten, which minimizes side effects in patients with celiac disease.

- Riomet, a liquid form of metformin (manufactured by Ranbaxy) in a dose of 500 mg/5 ml.

Guidelines for Getting Metformin

Taking metformin can be a bit tricky and sometimes requires a bit of fine-tuning by your doctor. Here are a few important tips from our clinical practice and research studies to make metformin "initiation" easy on you and your doctor:

- We always use what's called a "gradually escalating dosage schedule," starting with two tablets per day, half the anticipated final dose (see schedule A below); in patients with known gastrointestinal problems, we start with one tablet a day (see schedule B below).
- Starting low doses of metformin and increasing the number of pills gradually lets your body get used to metformin and lets us monitor any side effects carefully and adjust metformin dosage based on any that occur. It also dramatically decreases the likelihood of nausea or any other gastrointestinal side effects. (As is the case with all medications, side effects are very individual.)
- We prefer extended release ("XR") forms of metformin, which have fewer gastrointestinal side effects than does regular ("immediate-release") metformin.
- We usually start with generic metformin XR. It is covered by virtually all prescription plans and typically has a low or no copayment. So it's easier on both your stomach and your pocketbook!

The following guidelines for using metformin XR in the 500 mg dose may be helpful for your doctor. (We send this sheet to physicians who contact us regarding the dosage schedule.) Please read these instructions carefully, copy them as needed, and review them with your doctor before starting metformin.

Metformin Fact Sheet

Metformin is approved for the treatment of diabetes, and *other use is off label*.

Guidelines for Use

Take the medication twenty to thirty minutes before eating *or* with meals, as instructed. Follow one of the two schedules below as prescribed:

1. **Schedule A:** When first starting to take metformin, start with a total of **two tablets per day**—one at dinner and one at breakfast (or lunch if that's your first meal of the day). After one week, add a third tablet at dinner. After another week, add a fourth tablet at breakfast. **Do not increase the number of tablets at any time if you are having any stomach or other gastrointestinal side effects.**
2. **Schedule B:** If you are sensitive to medication or have gastrointestinal problems, start with one tablet at dinner and increase more gradually using the following schedule:

Day	Dosage Change	Total Tablets per Day
Day 8	Add a tab at breakfast	2
Day 15	Add another tab at dinner	3
Day 22	Add another tab at breakfast	4

3. If at any time you have serious stomach cramps, bad diarrhea, or gas pains, **stop the metformin completely for three days and then restart at half the dose you were taking when you got these symptoms.** Please call to let us know about these symptoms *or* if you have any questions regarding possible side effects. (A pill cutter can even be used to increase tabs more gradually if needed.) **New forms of metformin with fewer side effects are now available, but they cost more, so we do not prescribe them unless you have gastrointestinal side effects.**

Can I Take Metformin with Other Medications?

Most medications interact safely with metformin. However, always remind your physician what medicines you are taking and when there is a change in your medications. Don't forget that health supplements and other products you buy in a health-food store are "medications."

They can interact with physician-prescribed therapies and **can cause serious medical problems**, especially if your doctors are unaware that you are taking them.

What Are the Side Effects of Metformin?

Minor side effects: These side effects usually resolve after your body adjusts to taking the medicine for several weeks. These include mild diarrhea, nausea, or upset stomach. Taking metformin with meals can lessen these side effects. Call your physician if you experience severe discomfort or if the side effects last longer than several weeks.

Major side effects: Serious side effects are very rare and occur mostly in people who have kidney or liver dysfunction. The most serious side effect is lactic acidosis, which may be life threatening. Your physician will check your kidney and liver function to determine whether you are at risk.

Metformin's Downside

Most patients do well with metformin, but two types of side effects may occur. The first is common and involves the gastrointestinal tract. The other, called "lactic acidosis," is serious and extraordinarily rare (occurring in less than 1 in 32,000 cases of metformin use).

Side effects in the gastrointestinal tract may include:

- Nausea
- A metallic or odd taste in your mouth
- Upset stomach
- Diarrhea (which is the most common)

Gastrointestinal side effects can be reduced by using extended-release tablets and by taking metformin with meals. These side effects also resolve as your body adjusts to the medication, which is why we always start at a low dose and gradually increase the dosage.

Call your physician if you experience severe discomfort or if the side effects last longer than a few weeks.

Major Side Effects

Serious side effects are very rare and occur predominantly in people with significant kidney, liver, lung, or heart problems. This serious side effect, lactic acidosis, may be life threatening. Your physician will check your kidney function prior to prescribing metformin.

When to Discontinue Metformin Temporarily

Certain situations put you at risk for developing lactic acidosis. To reduce this risk, your physician may suggest you discontinue the medication under any of the following circumstances:

- You have surgery with general anesthesia.
- You have an X-ray procedure that requires the injection of a contrast dye (such as an MRI or a CT scan "with contrast").
- You have a severe dehydrating gastrointestinal illness (such as traveler's diarrhea, an intestinal virus, or food poisoning) with significant loss of body fluid due to severe vomiting, diarrhea, or an inability to keep fluids down.
- You are going to a party where you will be drinking more than two alcoholic beverages in two to three hours. **Excessive alcohol consumption should not be combined with any form of metformin.** Moderate alcohol, for example, one to two glasses of wine or beer in an evening, is okay.
- Note: You can stop the metformin "cold turkey" (without tapering it off) and restart it at the dose you were taking before you stopped.

Who should not take metformin:

- People who have kidney or liver abnormalities (unless your doctor thinks you have "fatty" liver disease—a disorder that is increasingly treated with metformin or other "insulin sensitizers")
- People who drink alcohol excessively
- People with serious medical conditions such as chronic cardiopulmonary disease or congestive heart failure

Not All Doctors Prescribe Metformin

Currently, metformin is *not* approved by the FDA for use as a weight-reduction drug. This means its use as a primary treatment for obesity is "off label." For that reason health care practitioners always advise our patients (and their legal guardians) in a written statement that treatment with metformin is "off label" (as noted in the Metformin Fact Sheet reproduced above).

Getting Metformin Covered

Metformin is available as a low-cost generic medication that costs far less than other FDA-approved anti-obesity agents, such as Meridia and Xenical. As with all medications, coverage depends on your prescription plan and the prescribing physician's treatment code.

Reimbursable diagnostic codes that your doctor can use, if applicable, include:

- Abnormal weight gain (251.1)
- Other hyperinsulinism (783.1)
- "Dysmetabolic" syndrome (277.7)

If you have Syndrome W, these codes accurately reflect your underlying medical condition and the manifestations of the syndrome. You may also have hypertension or abnormalities in cholesterol or other fats in your blood that have diagnostic codes. Check with a member of the clerical staff in your doctor's office to make sure that your physician codes your insurance information correctly.

Be a *Patient* Patient for Long-Term Success

One final comment before you take your first tablet: Because we go up slowly, you will *not* see the full effect of metformin in the first week or two. While you will see weight loss during this time, you have to wait to experience the total reduction in appetite and insulin levels until you are on the 1,500 mg- to 2,000 mg-per-day dose.

All other weight-reducing medications and diets give the highest rate of weight loss in early weeks, followed by a dramatic decline in weekly weight loss, with a plateau and a typical rebound in pounds after six months on the program. The slow start and progressive weight loss and that all-important absence of rebound are the key features of metformin and the Mogul Protocol that differ from all the other regimens.

Be patient. Remember that long-term goals are worth waiting and working for!

Chapter 13

ARE YOU SURE YOU DON'T
MEAN SYNDROME X?

Syndrome W by Any Other Name Is Not Syndrome X

NO, SYNDROME W IS *NOT* SYNDROME X! But left untreated, Syndrome W can progress to what has been called Syndrome X, or the metabolic syndrome, a later and more recognizable syndrome.

Most health-conscious men and women have heard of the metabolic syndrome, now estimated to affect more than 25 percent of all adults in the United States. That's a staggering number for a condition that's associated with almost all the disorders that cause early death in all industrialized nations: heart disease, diabetes, and cancer.

Syndrome X was defined originally in the late 1980s by famed endocrinologist Gerald Reaven, who called Syndrome X the "deadly quartet" of obesity, diabetes, hypertension, and lipid disturbances. And since his original publication, the metabolic syndrome has become the subject of countless research studies and publications by thousands of research groups worldwide.

Every day we see new information on the underlying molecular mechanisms and newest manifestations of this serious disorder. Amazingly, though, few treatments have been devised other than diet and exercise regimens, despite two decades of subsequent study.

Basically, Syndrome W is an early form of the important metabolic abnormality *insulin resistance*—a problem that often proceeds to the adult form of diabetes. **We chose to call it "W" to show that it's an** *alphabetical* and *chronological* antecedent to Syndrome X. The **W** represents the characteristic symptoms: weight gain, waist gain, and white-coat hypertension (blood pressure elevations in the doctor's office) in nondiabetic women with food cravings. All of these are early manifestations of insulin resistance that typically appear in perimenopause. What delays diagnosis, as noted in earlier chapters, is that the blood sugar tests of Syndrome W women are completely normal.

Calling an "X" an "X"

Two large committees standardized the definition of Syndrome X based on specific cutoff values for blood sugar, blood pressure, waist circumference, cholesterol, and triglycerides. You qualify for metabolic syndrome if you have three or more of these diagnostic criteria. Ironically, the most widely accepted definition of the metabolic syndrome (as initially defined by the National Cholesterol Education Program—the NCEP) has only one metabolic criterion: a fasting blood sugar greater than 110.

Amazingly, despite the metabolic syndrome's importance as a marker of underlying insulin resistance, insulin is not included in the current definition of the metabolic syndrome! Like most of you, most women with Syndrome W do *not* meet the current diagnostic criteria for the metabolic syndrome when we first see them in their forties, especially if they watch what they eat and exercise. Most women experience their first symptoms early in perimenopause, when they are early in the weight spiral. It's only after they "progress" farther down the insulin resistance pathway that full-fledged abnormalities develop; that's when they go from Syndrome W to Syndrome X.

The chart below compares the characteristics of the two syndromes. (The metabolic syndrome also includes HDL [good cholesterol] and triglyceride levels in the definition.) In this scheme of things, Syndrome W may be considered the "pre–metabolic syndrome." I prefer the term Syndrome W because it is so descriptive and highlights the fact that this is a phenomenon of women!

Defining Syndrome W

	Syndrome W	*Syndrome X*
Sugar	Normal	Fasting blood sugar $\geq$ 110
Insulin levels	Elevated	Not part of the definition
Weight	Weight gain $>$ twenty lbs. since the twenties	Not part of the definition
Waist	Waist gain more than two sizes	Waist circumference $\geq$ 35" in women Waist circumference $\geq$ 40" in men
Blood pressure (BP)	Single BP recording $>$ 140/85, two recordings of 130/85, or use of BP-lowering agent	Blood pressure $>$ 135/85
Appetite changes	Noticeable increase in appetite or new food cravings	Not part of the definition. Not considered relevant
Alternate name	The premetabolic syndrome	The metabolic syndrome

Part III

YOUR EATING PLAN:
Waist Management

Here you'll find everything you need to know about putting the Carb-Modified Diet to work. You get shortcuts, shopping techniques, grocery-store lists, and, best of all, solutions for the "sandwich generation"—women in their forties, fifties, and sixties who struggle to lose weight as they try to find time for an ever-expanding set of family responsibilities and workplace challenges. By the time you've read and absorbed the many great tips and ideas jam-packed into part III, living *la vida Mogul* will be practically second nature!

Chapter 14

HEAD START:
LAUNCHING THE MOGUL PROTOCOL

Getting the Show on the Road

OKAY, THINGS ARE GETTING INTERESTING! You've had the glucose tolerance test, found a physician to interpret your insulin curve and monitor your metformin, and now it's time to plunge forward into the Mogul Protocol. Clearly, this is an exciting milestone, a chance to jump-start progress. No more diets and exercise regimens that don't work. Now you have an extraordinarily effective way to overcome over-weight or obesity related to insulin resistance and hyperinsulinemia. But, remember, as noted by our first metformin patient, "**It only works if *you* work**." Make sure you can hit the ground running. Just take a few minutes to plot your course for starting and staying with the program.

Here are some important things to think about before you fill that prescription.

Know Thyself

Self-assessment is a critical first step to making meaningful changes. Here is our "Weight-Loss Readiness Questionnaire" to fine-tune that first step. Evaluate your life circumstances and consolidate your goals.

Answer these questions:

1. **Are you prepared to make dietary changes that promote weight loss and lifelong weight control?**

2. **Do you have the support of people you're with on a daily basis?**
3. **Why do you want to lose weight? Select ones that apply:**

   - Health needs (reducing cholesterol, blood pressure level, blood sugar)
   - Health benefits (prevention of abnormalities in blood pressure, cholesterol, and blood sugar)
   - Family health history of diabetes, heart disease, or high blood pressure
   - Increased mobility
   - Improved performance of daily activities (doing housework; shopping; sitting comfortably on trains, on planes, in movies)
   - Improved appearance and self-image

4. **Is the timing right? Look at your current workload, social life, and stress level, and figure out whether this is a good time to start and stay on a weight-loss program.**

The last of these questions is the first one we ask because it goes right to the heart of the matter of making any eating plan stick (and work).

5. **Assess your readiness factor. Will you have some time to devote to your diet each day?** It's important to make a realistic appraisal. Can you really free up a little time each day to change your eating and exercise? You may not think this is the best time to make a big commitment to lifestyle changes if you're starting a new job, moving to a new city, or dealing with any other new stressful life event (divorce, separation, death or illness of a parent, mate, or child). If you're doubtful, consider postponing the start-up date. Finding the right time to launch your new efforts will make the program more likely to succeed.

   Medication should be reserved for serious weight-loss efforts and integrated into a comprehensive lifestyle program. Metformin can be a miracle for a motivated dieter, but it's not a quick fix, and it doesn't work without other changes in diet and lifestyle. Be brutally honest with yourself, and you can avoid the frustration of having to put the plan on hold while you deal with a life-threatening illness or an unanticipated stressor. On the other hand, if your response is, "This is as good a time as ever," your nonanswer probably signals future success. You understand that weight management is time management. When you have Syndrome W, time is truly your enemy, and you don't want to waste another day.

6. **What are your weight-loss goals in pounds and clothing size?** Consider short-term as well as long-term goals. Think about how great you'll feel after you downsize by just one size. Approach your weight-loss odyssey in management mode—ideally, even at the micromanagement level. Take stock of your assets:

   - What are your options for shopping and meal preparation?
   - What support system is available to help you free up time to shop for healthy foods and prepare breakfasts and take-away lunches, to exercise and participate in weight-friendly activities (yoga, meditation, relaxation)?
   - Think about liabilities that loom ahead. What about dietary preferences (yours and your family's)? Dietary constraints (lactose intolerance or irritable bowel problems)?
   - Factor in your budget and recognize that you may need to get up earlier or go to bed later to get the extra half hour you need to get it all done.

Forget the Quick Fix

Throw out your low-fat staples and all calorically dense and sugar-laden foods in your house. If you can't bring yourself to throw food away, donate all expendables (candies, cookies, cakes, cereals) to community shelters. Just get them out of your house and out of your life. This is a service to your whole family. Next, go on a shopping trip to restock with fresh and frozen vegetables and fruits; low-fat dairy products, such as yogurt with Equal (aspartame) or Splenda (sucralose), cottage cheese, no-sugar-added ice cream and frozen bars, skim or 1 percent milk; soups; turkey; chicken; low-fat deli meats; eggs and egg substitutes; veggie burgers; reduced-fat cheeses; diet salad dressings; and on and on. If you have time to assemble meals or do some modular cooking (see chapter 18), add to your shopping list fresh herbs, vegetable stock, canned tomatoes, olive oil, flavored vinegars, mustards, and jarred sauces (nonsweetened teriyaki, salsa).

Just make sure you leave behind trigger foods and any of the newly minted, overprocessed, low-carb wonders that are replacing the low-fat Oreos of old.

Set Realistic Goals

It's hard to be thin (after adolescence when fat-storing hormones surge), and you don't have to be. Every study shows that a 10 percent weight loss promotes health, prevents type 2 diabetes, and reduces the risk of heart disease.

After one year, the average weight loss in patients who stay with our program (the 80 percent who return for two or more visits) is close to 15 percent, and many make it into the 25 percent range, shedding forty-plus pounds. Metformin expands your food choices, and the Carb-Modified Diet isn't strict or boring like many other food regimens. So you can relax, steady your mind, and move ahead with confidence, knowing that this time, the pounds you shed will be gone forever.

Slow Down to Speed Up:
Smell the Roses, Taste the Grapes

We Americans eat too quickly. The brisk pace of contemporary society and the availability of fast food have created a generation of children weaned on Chicken McNuggets, Double Whoppers, and Taco Bell treats. The duration of the average meal at fast-food establishments that serve these entrees is less than ten minutes—far fewer than necessary for "satiety," studies tell us. Obesity specialists frequently refer to availability, palatability, and portion size as major causes of the current obesity crisis.

I believe it's also about the pace at which we eat. If we slow down and actually taste some of those fast-food specials, we might detect the flavor—mostly salt or sugar—and discern the blandness of the beef, the chicken, or the cheese that it camouflages. Today, there's a trend called the slow food movement, which is an international response to the frenetic pace of the American eating style. Its aficionados favor a return to fresh fruits and vegetables, non-mass-produced (artisanal) breads and cheeses, and lovingly prepared simple foods in the traditions of the fare of farm folk from Sicily, Crete, Berkeley (California), the Berkshires (Massachusetts), and the Hudson River Valley (New York). Truly, food is one of the great joys in life, and you should fuss over it and savor it whenever possible.

My mother was a fantastic and creative cook with a heavy hand on fat. She added butter or cheese to almost everything, and her food was incredibly tasty, in addition to being calorie laden. Her ideas of vegetables were cauliflower with burnt butter (now *beurre noisette*), creamed carrots (with white sauce made from cream), and deep-fried eggplant topped with fresh mozzarella or *viennoise*. When she bought pizza, she would order extra cheese and then top it with shredded Vermont cheddar and extra-aged, imported-only parmesan (long before *quattro formaggio* became a household word).

While my mother trimmed the extra fat off baked Virginia ham (before studding the neatly cut diamonds with cloves) and brisket (before browning it with garlic and onions), she bought only prime, well-marbled steaks, and corned beef, tongue, and smoked salmon with visible fat interspersed between the darker red fibers. She recognized and taught her offspring that fat did indeed add flavor. (Fortunately, she also stressed the virtues of exercise to counterbalance our gluttony.)

Nonetheless, Mom was very fussy about food. She never ate anything she didn't like, and she never made us kids "finish everything" on our plates because of underfed children from some starving nation. Thus, my brother and I developed not only an appreciation of great food but a few helpful habits along the way.

Learn about Loving Food and Losing Weight

You may be surprised to hear that many people actually gain weight by eating foods they dislike. This may seem paradoxical, but I've had many patients report that they often continue to eat simply because they aren't satisfied with what they've eaten.

Resolve that if you don't like it, you won't eat it. Understand that consuming calories from food you don't care for often leads to overeating, in an endless and elusive search for something that satisfies. If your food doesn't please you, you'll probably continue to eat to turn off the "appetite" switch (somewhat different from the hunger switch).

Consider the Food Experiences of These Women

Carla's Cookies

Carla had always loved to bake. As she began to lose weight, she changed her baking habits. She began to bake for others at the office. She started to bring in big batches of chocolate-chip cookies, brownies, blondies, or lemon squares for her mostly male and under-forty coworkers whose metabolisms could more easily tolerate these densely caloric products of her evening activities. In the weeks before Christmas one year, Carla saw her weight-loss efforts go astray for the first time in months. She told me that she didn't know why she was gaining weight. "Nothing has changed. I'm still following the diet program." But her own tale of baking gave us the answer: "I may be eating a few more cookies than I used to after my nightly baking sprees. Come to think of it, I finished almost half a pan of brownies last night. They just didn't come out like they usually do—none of that fudge taste where one is all you need. So I just kept tasting them to figure out what went wrong with the recipe. Amazing . . . I didn't even like them and I kept eating them. I never eat more than one when they come out right."

Marcy's Mousse

Marcy, one of my most recalcitrant patients and a very busy nurse, lived alone, worked long hours, and then went home and ate "whatever was around" and especially "a lot after dinner." She took metformin, attended nutrition/behavior workshops, and modified her diet, but for months the scale barely budged.

Though disappointed with her weight-loss progress, Marcy kept a good attitude and remained committed to making the lifestyle changes she knew she needed to get her insulin levels under control. I was sure that she had succeeded when, during a follow-up visit, she gave me an annotated recipe (see below) for the dessert that kept her from eating all night long, like she used to.

Her recipe went like this:

"I take one-half ounce of Baker's unsweetened chocolate and melt it in the microwave; then I mix in a little Splenda and let it cool down a bit. I take a few heaping tablespoons of low-fat Cool-Whip—maybe one-half cup—and blend it into the chocolate, but I don't overmix it because the different textures and the flecks of chocolate add a nice touch."

Clearly, Marcy had learned how to use all of her senses to eat and enjoy a single dessert item. Savoring one great, calorically controlled treat warded off an evening's worth of mindless eating. For her, it was the key behavioral change that ratcheted up her weight loss, which was now more than 15 percent of her baseline weight.

Don't Be a Grabber or a Gulper

You need to eat slowly to feel full and satisfied. This reduces overeating after mealtime. Make a point of tasting and enjoying each mouthful. Follow these hints for slowing down your consumption to speed up your weight loss.

Don't Grab Food on Your Way out the Door

If you have a tendency to grab, gulp, wolf, or snarf, you're going to need some radical shifts in eating style. You will have to alter the way you eat for long-term weight maintenance. Know that you need to slow down to taste what you're eating. Figure out how to have a real lunch and a real dinner—times when you actually sit down for at least twenty minutes to eat and enjoy food. Try to avoid the habit of nibbling at your desk or wolfing down a Whopper on the way to a meeting. Keep an apple in your backpack or an orange in your briefcase.

If you simply can't make the time to eat right, substitute a snack of fruit or a beverage rather than backsliding to bad eating that will then require an overhaul. You can always sip a Diet Coke or an extra-hot low-fat latte. (It's hard to drink carbonated or hot beverages on the run. They *make* you slow down.)

You don't have to do all of these things perfectly at the start, but do try to increase your awareness of destructive eating habits. That will lead you to develop constructive substitutes. You've probably been eating for more than a quarter of a century, so you won't change your comfy habits overnight. And that's okay. Be gentle with yourself; just look for progress—slow, steady baby steps.

Take a Sensory Overload Approach

When rating wines, wine tasters look at the color and clarity and describe the aroma and nose of the grape. That twenty-six-ounce wineglass lets you put your nose in the glass and smell the bouquet. Today, thicker and smaller black wineglasses are the newest wine toys, designed to allow wine connoisseurs to discern and separate visual and olfactory from taste factors.

Also take a good look at what you're eating. If you see grease on the surface of the soup or oil staining the paper wrapper or swimming in the bottom of the Mexican-food take-out container, just say no. Don't eat it! Looking at food can help you figure out what you should and shouldn't eat.

Dissect Individual Tastes

Learn what you really like to eat. This is a little like learning to hear the string section in a symphony or to note the folds of fabric in a portrait rather than just viewing an artistic work as a whole. This process takes a little training but yields great dividends. Extra sensory input enhances the total experience and satiety at the brain. Try this when dining with friends, and you may be surprised at the results.

I've had a few of these eating epiphanies myself. In fact, a great dinner my first night in Vail, Colorado, actually triggered this section. I ate pecan-crusted walleye that was true perfection, a lesson in simple yet complex cuisine and exquisite presentation: crunchy, pecan-coated, moist, perfectly cooked, enamel-white, freshwater pike atop a bed of fresh-from-the-garden, al dente, steamed baby string beans, and lemon-infused roasted fingerling potato hash, accompanied by basil-dusted grape tomato halves. It was truly heaven, and I enjoyed every slow, flavor-filled moment and easily skipped dessert. The entrée reflected many of the Mogul Protocol's principles—a colorful enactment of the Carb-Modified Diet and the role of food presentation. For me, it was also an example of how slow food leads to weight loss when, several days later, I discovered my ski pants were considerably looser.

Now that you have the overview, it's time to move from "mind" to "matter."

Chapter 15

FIVE EASY PIECES
AND THE 4-3-2-1 PYRAMID

If This Is Tuesday, It Must Be Tuna:
The Structured Meal Plan

YOU BASICALLY NEED ONLY TWO CONCEPTS to lose weight on the Mogul Protocol—five easy pieces and the 4-3-2-1 pyramid.

The 4-3-2-1 pyramid is new, but the "pieces" have been around and in use since 1974. The original version was developed at Barnard College to help students lose the infamous "freshman ton," the ten to twenty pounds that each freshman girl gains after leaving the fold of family life for the freedom of carb-loaded dormitory food in an all-you-can-eat environment. It consisted of a set of instructions on how to navigate food lines to develop lifelong eating patterns to overcome overweight and promote health, and this diet embodied all the principles I use today:

- Avoiding densely caloric sugars and fats
- Consuming lots of low-fat protein, vegetables, and fruits
- Eating low-fat dairy products
- Indulging in that all-important occasional treat to eliminate deprivation

I believed then (as I believe now) that this approach was preferable to the on-again, off-again "diet" of the month for helping women avoid the weight extremes that characterized college campuses. I had learned early on, after just a few months of working with overweight students, that even the most highly motivated college women did not shed pounds with traditional diets. So I'd switched tactics to what I've continued to use in a lifetime of helping women with long-term weight management.

I told Barnard women then (as I tell women today) when they asked for a copy of "my diet," that there's no magic in the handouts that spell out the virtues of those low-fat proteins and vegetables. I instructed them to spend extra time at the salad bar (with low-calorie dressing); to ask for a double serving of the meat entrée sans the starches and the sauce; to take an extra apple back to their rooms; and to walk resolutely past the dessert table, looking neither to the left nor the right. That was then and this is now, but the rules have not changed.

This is still my diet philosophy: a set of simple-to-use rules.

The 4-3-2-1 pyramid and the five easy pieces are spin-offs of the thirty-five-year-old Barnard Diet. The pyramid was created to take the program public in response to requests from nutritionists and doctors in our community.

I am not a fan of superstructured diets that dictate each day's menu: "If this is Tuesday, it must be tuna." I believe the lifestyle change we advocate involves figuring out what to eat and when. The materials used in our clinic and shared with colleagues are the tools we use. You must create your own menus and meal plans based on your own food preferences, schedule, and living situations. That's the only way you can "own" and follow a new eating plan for a lifetime.

Here are (a) the five easy pieces, (b) the 4-3-2-1 pyramid (as published in the medical literature), and (c) the exact materials we give patients (and physicians) to make our program user friendly and clear.

Five Easy Pieces

1. No free (added) sugars: no candy, cookies, cake, or cereal
2. No starches (refined carbohydrates), bread, cereal, rice, or pasta until 4 p.m.
3. Vegetables for breakfast, lunch, dinner, and in between
4. Lots of fish, chicken, other low-fat protein foods, and high-fiber (low-glycemic-index) fruits
5. Low-fat dairy and fruit desserts to avoid deprivation

For long-term weight loss, remember that it's the timing and the quality of the carbs and protein you eat. Keep it simple. Follow the foolproof food pyramid for healthy weight loss forever.

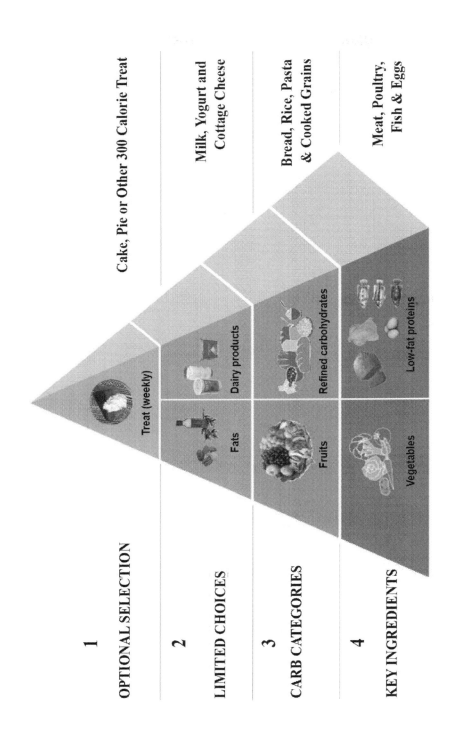

1
OPTIONAL SELECTION
Cake, Pie or Other 300 Calorie Treat

2
LIMITED CHOICES
Milk, Yogurt and Cottage Cheese

3
CARB CATEGORIES
Bread, Rice, Pasta & Cooked Grains

4
KEY INGREDIENTS
Meat, Poultry, Fish & Eggs

Treat (weekly)

Fats   Dairy products

Fruits   Refined carbohydrates

Vegetables   Low-fat proteins

Summary of the Mogul Pyramid

**4 servings of low-fat protein
(~100 calories)**
3 oz cooked fish, skinned poultry
low-fat ground poultry or beef
eggs or beans in equal calorie amounts

3 servings of fruit (~100 calories)
1 medium piece of fruit,
1 cup berries
No fruit juice or dried fruits
Choose low glycemic index
fruits!

**2 servings of fat
(~200–300 calories/day)**
Olive oil, butter, margarine
(read labels)
Cheese—100–120 cal/oz
Nuts—½ oz or
2 tablespoons
Avocado—½ small

4 servings of vegetables (MINIMUM)
½ cup cooked or raw vegetables
1 cup raw leafy greens

**3 servings of starches (~100 calories)
MUST BE LATER IN THE DAY!**
high fiber or multigrain
when possible
1 oz bread, 2 slices low-cal bread
½ cup cooked pasta, rice, beans

**2 servings low-fat dairy
(80–120 calories)**
8 oz skim milk = 6 oz
1% milk = 4 oz 2% milk
½ cup low- or no-fat
cottage cheese
1 low-calorie sugar-free
ice cream bar
1 6–8 oz low-fat,
low-calorie yogurt

**1 weekly treat (after the first month:
~300–350 calories)**
SMALL piece cake, pie, or portion of dessert

Each serving is about 100 calories (80 to 120), with the exception of vegetables, which are typically about 50 calories per cup. *These are per-day maximums of each food group except veggies, of which you're allowed six or more servings a day.*

With the pyramid, you get an easy way to stay within a total number of calories per day, and this leads to weight loss of one to two pounds per week. No need to count calories every time you take a bite!

The pyramid provides:

- A balance of healthy foods
- Lots of choices
- No dietary extremes of low-carbohydrate and low-fat diets

It's fine to mix and match (exchange a fruit for a milk serving), but just stay within the five easy pieces philosophy. This is an eating plan for life, so tailor it to your own individual food preferences and lifestyle, and it will work for you. (Read all materials to gain a thorough understanding.)

The only caveat: You have to know a serving, memorize a serving, and stick with a serving! It consists of about 100 calories (a range of 80 to 120). See the following details on average servings.

Protein Servings: Four per Day

One serving equals:

> Three ounces fish, seafood, skinless chicken, or turkey
> Two to three ounces lean beef, veal, or pork
> Two ounces ultralean (maximum 7 percent fat) ground beef or veal
> Two to three ounces turkey deli meat, turkey sausage, or turkey bacon
> Three ounces low-fat ground turkey or chicken
> One-half cup legumes or beans
> One-half cup cottage cheese or low-fat yogurt (count as a dairy *or* a protein serving)

Note: Keep in mind that fatty fishes (salmon, fresh tuna, bluefish, swordfish, herring, and other dark-meat fishes) have extra fat calories. These also have many health benefits, such as improving the balance of fats in the bloodstream. Just remember that they're high in calories, which means that consuming very big portions will slow your weight loss. Follow these tips:

- Learn to estimate portion size of fish, and stay within the total servings per day guidelines above.
- Trim all visible fat and skin from meat, poultry, and fish.

Fruit Servings: Three per Day

Know what counts as a fruit serving. Know that all fruits are not equal.

What Counts as a Fruit Serving?

You get about seventy to one hundred calories from one medium-size piece of fresh fruit or its equivalent (two fresh apricots or small plums), so there's your fruit serving.

Other fruit info that can help:

- Small fruits like berries are high in fiber and low in glycemic index and calories and have about sixty to eighty calories per cup.
- Cherries, grapes, cut-up melons, and unsweetened fresh fruits are about one hundred calories per cup.
- Unlike other highly dense caloric foods, an extra one-half cup of berries or other low- to medium-glycemic-index fruits won't deter weight loss.

All Fruits Are Not Equal

Differences relate to each fruit's glycemic index (GI). The GI is a measure of how rapidly your blood sugar rises after eating carbohydrates.

Low-glycemic-index fruits are an important part of the Carb-Modified Diet. You can eat three servings a day. Eat your fruit at breakfast, lunch, dinner, 4 p.m. snack, or late-night snack. Low-glycemic-index fruits are the only carbohydrates allowed at breakfast and lunch. The lists make it easy to choose the right fruits for your eating plan.

Best fruits:

Citrus: orange, grapefruit, tangerine, clementine
Berries: all are low-cal and low-glycemic-index

Worst fruits (eat these fruits occasionally; mix them in a fruit salad with citrus and other low-glycemic-index fruits):

Banana: avoid those that are very ripe
Pineapple
Other tropical fruits, such as mango and papaya
Grapes
Watermelon

In between (one piece is your recommended serving size unless noted otherwise):

Apricots (two to three)

Apple (small)

Cherries (one cup = twenty to thirty cherries)

Melons (These vary a great deal—the glycemic index depends on the source and the ripeness.)

Peaches

Pears

Plums (one large or two to three small)

Nectarines

Fruit Rules

- Fruit juices are not allowed.
- Avoid all dried fruits (especially raisins, dried cranberries, dates, and "preserved" tropical fruits).

For more on glycemic index, see the books by Jennie Brand Miller (*The Glucose Revolution, The GI Factor*), the book *Good Carbs, Bad Carbs*, by Johanni Burani, and these websites: www.mendosa.com, www.glycemicindex.com, j.brandmiller@biochem.usyd.edu.au.

Starch Servings: Three per Day

Make sure you choose high-fiber, low-glycemic-index starches, such as whole-grain bread, brown rice, quinoa, and other whole grains. Choose whole-wheat pasta or pasta made from whole durum wheat over other kinds, including soy pasta, which is pricey and often unpalatable. If you have gluten intolerance or celiac disease, now diagnosed in one of every hundred Americans, you should select one of the new oat- or rice-based pastas.

One starch serving equals:

One ounce bread, hard roll, or bagel (Do note that most bagels are five ounces each!)

Two slices low-calorie or "light" or "diet" bread (forty to fifty calories per slice)

One "light" (ninety-calorie) English muffin

One-half cup rice, pasta, beans, or corn

One small baked potato (eight ounces)

One-half sweet potato or yam (four to six ounces)

Carb Rules

Eat no breakfast cereals for breakfast or lunch.

Remember that even high-fiber cereals and oatmeal are off-limits for breakfast. If you have Syndrome W, you have an elevated insulin response curve, which means that even high-fiber breakfast food will trigger an insulin response. If you really miss your oatmeal or need fiber for "regularity," eat a bowl of oatmeal as your 4 p.m. snack. Just make sure you choose rolled oats, not instant or quick-cooking oats.

Oatmeal once a week is okay, but for long-term weight maintenance, you need to find other foods to eat and reduce your reliance on oatmeal and other high-fiber, whole-grain breakfast foods. This can be a major stumbling block for many people until they notice that their favorite high-fiber cereal made a difference—they didn't feel as well as when they ate one of the other breakfast options. And on days that they ate the old favorites, they did find themselves much hungrier. I'm an empiricist (driven by observation), so I would encourage you to go ahead, experiment, and see for yourself. Just try not to venture too far from camp.

Save sandwiches for dinner.

While whole-grain breads are certainly better than breads made from overprocessed wheat flours, they're still carbs and cause a spike in insulin levels. **The key to the Carb-Modified Diet is to postpone starches until later in the day. Soup and salad work well for people who try this approach. This is an important change that's necessary for your long-term success.** Have your main meal at lunch instead of dinner if you prefer. Just keep starches off your plate and pile it with low-fat protein and lots of veggies. Sample the bounty of great soups and protein-rich salads and vegetable entrees.

Not sure about this? See how many people nod off at work during afternoon meetings. Check out what the nappers ate for lunch. Truth is, it's easy to wind up supersluggish an hour after eating an otherwise healthy pita wrap. So get off the sandwich kick altogether and move on to healthier eating. You'll have much less downtime in the afternoon.

Dairy Products: Two per Day (80–110 Calories Each)

One dairy serving equals:

Eight ounces skim milk = six ounces of 1 percent milk = four ounces of 2 percent milk and total eighty to a hundred calories. Because whole milk is high in fat, you should use it sparingly.

Six- to eight-ounce container of low-fat yogurt with Equal (aspartame) or Splenda (sucralose)

One-half to one cup cottage cheese (low-fat)

One low-calorie, low-fat, no-sugar-added frozen ice cream or yogurt bar

One-third cup no-sugar-added low-fat ice cream or frozen yogurt

To increase your choices, count yogurt and cottage cheese as either proteins or breakfast dairy selections.

Fat Servings: Two per Day (200–300 Calories Total)

Eat fats in moderation.

Monounsaturated fats, such as olive oil, are best. Avoid trans fats, which increase your risk of heart disease. Peanut oil, walnut oil, corn oil, and safflower oil are good for their health benefits. Use the guidelines below:

Oils:	1 teaspoon oil = 40 calories; 1 tablespoon = 120 calories
Mayonnaise:	1 tablespoon mayonnaise = 100 calories; "light" or "diet" mayo = 40–60 calories/tablespoon
Butter:	1 pat butter = 50 calories (1 teaspoon = 33 calories)

Margarines and "lite" margarines vary (read labels).

Salad dressings:	Regular (nondiet) dressings vary from 100 to 120 calories/tablespoon, depending on fat and sugar content.
"Light" or "diet" dressings:	Range from 0 to 50 calories/tablespoon. You don't have to count the dressings in this category if

the calorie content is 30 or less and if you don't exceed 1 ounce (2 tablespoons) per serving.

Cheese (Read labels on "nondairy" [e.g., tofu cheeses] and yogurt cheeses):

Regular cheeses	90–120 calories/ounce (average 100 calories/ounce)
Low-fat cheeses	Typically 80–100 calories/ounce
No-fat cheeses	Rarely edible
Other Fat Exchanges:	½ ounce nuts 1 ounce (two thin slices) bacon (crisp only) ½ a small avocado 1½ ounces (3 tablespoons) hummus

Fat Rules

Eat no nuts if they're your nemesis.

Nuts are increasingly advocated, as new research studies demonstrate their health benefits. Nonetheless, for many people, nuts are high on the list of trigger foods. If you love nuts, limit your purchases to four-ounce packages (or keep them off your shelves completely) to avoid overindulging in this calorically dense fat option. Choose nuts like walnuts and almonds, unsalted and unadulterated. Walnut and peanut oil can also provide health benefits.

Salad dressings, sauces:

Don't use if the calorie content exceeds forty calories per tablespoon. Read labels for fat (and sugar) content.

Weekly Treat: One Per Week

(You get a treat a week after the first month or your loss of the first five pounds.)

Enjoy your 300- to 350-calorie option! Select a small piece of cake, pie, or portion of dessert. Examples include:

Half of a three-inch-square brownie
One-sixth of a ten-inch-diameter fruit pie
One-eighth of a cream-based pie
Small (1½-inch) wedge of cheesecake

Small chocolate ice-cream sundae
One-half cup crème brûlée
Two-thirds cup berry crisp or fruit cobbler

Make sure your weekly treat doesn't morph into a daily treat. Keep any trigger foods—temptations you can't resist—off your list.

Detailing Other Options

Liquids

Drink eight glasses of liquids each day: water, coffee, tea, but limit diet soda and diet iced tea to three per day maximum.

Spices and Condiments

Use to add flavor to your diet. Rubs and mixtures are great time-savers that can dress up vegetables, chicken, fish, and egg dishes. Most condiments are okay in moderation. Use honey mustard and ketchup sparingly, and when you do use them, check out the sugar, fat, and calorie content.

Sodium

According to today's dietary recommendations, Americans should reduce their salt intake. Eliminating highly processed foods and avoiding fast-food eateries are the way to go, because many of the available products are both supersized and supersaturated with salt. Moderation is a good idea. Many African American men and women are especially salt sensitive, which increases their risk of developing high blood pressure. However, one of the actions of insulin on the kidneys is to increase the amount of salt and water you retain. So if you have Syndrome W and you're just starting the Mogul Protocol, you'll decrease bloating if you avoid excess dietary salt.

By decreasing insulin levels, metformin may help to diminish your salt retention. Once again, as with carbs, this expands your food choices. You will discover that a little salt restriction can go a long way. But severe restriction is rarely necessary—plus, it makes food taste bland and unappealing. Do choose lower-sodium soups, vegetable juices, and prepared foods—and spare the saltshaker (don't put it on the table).

Logging Off

The Carb-Modified Diet portion of the Mogul Protocol works simply with metformin to treat the cause of weight gain associated with Syndrome W. **Metformin dramatically increases dietary options for women with insulin elevations. These options are otherwise off-limits on other low-carbohydrate diets that require severe carbohydrate restriction to keep insulin surges at bay.**

Take advantage of metformin's ability to reduce appetite and eliminate insulin spikes and expand your dietary choices to a wide range of fresh fruits and vegetables, low-fat proteins, and low-fat dairy products. Supplement these with our suggestions for alternatives to fat- and calorie-loaded snacks and desserts.

Now, for the very first time ever, you can avoid deprivation and boredom and control your weight with an eating plan with ample choices and diet variety. You can easily individualize the 4-3-2-1 pyramid to your dietary preferences and schedule demands. The "one-size-fits-all" mentality of most diets just doesn't work for most people and probably has not worked for you. The materials used in our clinic will explain exactly what you need to do. These tips have helped hundreds of women with Syndrome W reach their goal weight and stay there year after year when they return for follow-up visits.

Our handouts (in chapter 23) are the results of countless conversations with women who have used the Mogul Protocol to overcome Syndrome W cravings and weight gain. You can join these women in becoming healthier as your own insulin levels decline with correctly targeted medication and a diet that lets you eat almost anything and everything you've ever wanted.

Have fun as you shift the contents of your supermarket cart and your cupboards. Dieting, like eating, is a creative process. You can still love food and lose weight if you shop and cook carefully.

Chapter 16

SOLUTIONS FOR THE SANDWICH GENERATION

Indispensable Differences Weigh In

The five easy pieces boil down to two big basic changes: breakfast and lunch. These are the keys to success—the essential elements of the Carb-Modified Diet that differentiate it from other "healthy" balanced dietary regimens.

Now let's go through the day and learn the drill to make these simple but seminal changes to lose weight and keep it off forever. As flexible as our food plan is, these changes are not negotiable. They are absolute and essential aspects of the dietary regimen.

Here's what you have to do:

- Eliminate carbs at breakfast.
- Give up sandwiches of all kinds at lunch.
- Get on the soup-and-salad bandwagon at lunch instead.

I believe this is a small price to pay for the pleasure and potential benefits of permanent weight loss. Remember, this is not a diet—it's a lifestyle change.

#1—Breakfast: Bite the Bullet, Not the Banana

If you have Syndrome W and you're serious about losing weight, the first thing you need to do is fix breakfast.

You need to find a substitute for the muffins, bagels, doughnuts, and cereal that are parts of the American way. The major dietary change in our program is breakfast, and it's a hard game to change in the United States, where, more than in any other nation, breakfast is a high-carbohydrate event.

Add to this the current size of a bagel—five ounces, which translates to one carb serving per ounce of bagel—and the availability and consumption of bagels in the United States, the popularity and speed with which Americans eat doughnuts, croissants, muffins, and Pop-Tarts, and you'll probably have an explanation for much of the obesity epidemic.

In order to lose weight and keep it off, you need to find alternate foods for breakfast or skip it until later in the morning. Substituting a rasher of bacon or a cheese omelet is not a reasonable alternative.

Fact #6 (in chapter 19) explains it all. The results of this landmark rigorously controlled study of test meals conducted at the Harvard Clinical Research Center showed unequivocally that what you eat for breakfast determines how many calories you'll consume later in the day. (The study showed a statistically significant difference in afternoon—noon to 6 p.m.—caloric consumption when study subjects ate scrambled eggs, whole-grain oats, or instant oatmeal at breakfast.)

If you have Syndrome W and an abnormal sugar-stimulated insulin curve (definitive hyperinsulinemia), your afternoon intake will increase if you eat carbs (other than fruit) at breakfast, just like it did for those overweight, nondiabetic adolescents in the Harvard study. The more sugar and higher-glycemic load of carbs you eat at breakfast, the hungrier you'll be, and the more you'll eat in the hours that follow. Metformin helps you control your breakfast-related insulin spikes, but it can't eliminate them entirely.

Remember, even healthy high-fiber, whole-oat cereal will make you eat more throughout the day than if you had started the morning with a plate of simple scrambled eggs. Fiber One and any of the "carb-controlled cereals" from health-food stores and drugstores are no better. Even the highest-fiber, whole-grain cereal is off-limits except as an occasional option—about once a week after the first month of weight loss. Frosted flakes and other sugar-coated cereals are verboten forever!

Breaking out of the Breakfast Mold

To come up with your own ideal breakfast, check out sample meals on page 95. Find out what you like and "make it your own." There are fifty ways to cook an omelet/frittata/"scramble." If you hate eggs, go with other options.

Figure out whether you want variety or you prefer the same meal. There are lots of choices, but the first choice you need to make is whether you want to eat a variety of breakfasts or whether you prefer having only one. You, like many of my patients and nutritionist colleagues, may find that you prefer a single breakfast solution. After following hundreds of women (and quite a few adolescents and men), I've observed that in contrast to other meals, where variety is helpful, the same breakfast Monday through Friday, day in and day out, works well for most of my highly successful patients.

Of all the meals in the day, breakfast is the one you're most likely to grab on the way out the door. That it is the "most important meal of the day," instilled in all of us as children, may be scientifically correct, but it just doesn't address the realities of most contemporary women (and men).

The first hour of the day is a busy time for most women. If your early-morning scenario resembles a marathon, change your breakfast ritual, preferably into a single selection (or one alternate choice) on the weekdays. Then, like the large number of long-term success stories in our practice, stay with what works and try not to stray.

When you need to be on autopilot in the a.m. you'll need to do some heavy-duty planning. Make a berry-yogurt smoothie or crustless quiche the night before. Pop a portion into the microwave or eat it at room temperature.

Put an orange and no-sugar-added yogurt in your briefcase or backpack. Whether it's a low-fat latte (the tastiest and most available version of the liquid-protein diet) or an apple and a small chunk of cheese or hardboiled eggs to take on the train (a favorite of many commuters and early-morning carpoolers), do whatever works for you. Just remember to bypass the muffins and bagels at Dunkin' Donuts and the scones at Starbucks if you stop for coffee on the way to work or school.

When you do limit your a.m. carbs, it's worlds easier to avoid overeating at lunch, dinner, and in between.

The New Breakfast

You're leaving behind the high-carb breakfast for a new way. Choose one of the options listed here, and add one fruit with a low glycemic index (berries, orange, or grapefruit). Drink coffee, tea, water, or diet soda.

- Vegetable omelet. Spray a nonstick pan with vegetable spray. Create a three-egg-white omelet with fresh eggs, Egg Beaters, or an egg-white-only product; add ½ to 1 cup mixed vegetables (onions, mushrooms, pepper, tomatoes, spinach, etc.). Also, you may want to toss in a little low-fat ham (1 to 2 ounces) or cheese (½ to 1 ounce) for variety once or twice a week.
- Vegetable "scramble." Use any of the omelet ingredients, but cook the vegetables or low-fat ham first, then add the eggs, and cook to the desired doneness. Remove the pan from the heat, sprinkle on shredded cheese (if desired), cover for a minute to let it melt, and serve.
- Crustless quiche or frittata. Use any combo of vegetables used in your omelet and scramble. Make in advance and reheat in the microwave.
- Scrambled eggs. Use one whole egg and two egg whites or all egg whites with two slices of turkey bacon, Canadian bacon, low-fat turkey sausage, or extra-lean ham.
- Yogurt. Choose 6- to 8-ounce container low-fat yogurt sweetened with Equal (aspartame) or Splenda (sucralose).
- Yogurt smoothie. Simply blend 1 cup plain nonfat yogurt with 1 cup berries and some Splenda or Equal. Eat with a spoon. Do not overblend or liquefy. This should be the consistency of thick soup.
- Cottage cheese Danish. Mix cottage cheese with cinnamon and sugar substitute (Splenda tastes best). Spread on a single slice of toasted low-calorie (40 calories per slice) whole-wheat bread or crisp apple slices that have been cored but not peeled. Place in a toaster oven under the broiler for a minute or two to melt the topping.
- English muffin mound. Have this no more than once a week. Use a low-calorie or "light" ninety-calorie muffin or half of a large English muffin. Whole-grain is best. Add whole scrambled eggs, egg whites, or Egg Beaters. Layer any of the following:
  - Canadian bacon or turkey ham slice
  - Turkey bacon or turkey sausage (split lengthwise after cooking)

- Slice of low-fat cheddar, Swiss, or provolone cheese
- Smear of low-fat goat or herb cream cheese (best when spread directly on muffin)
- Slice of tomato
- Drained salsa, chopped chiles, or olives

Breakfasts for a Week

Monday

Yogurt smoothie with blueberries

Blend 1 cup blueberries with 1 to 1½ cups nonfat vanilla or plain yogurt sweetened to taste (Equal or Splenda). Add three ice cubes to the blender for a thicker shake if you plan to drink this immediately after you make it.

Tuesday

Red pepper, spinach, and goat cheese "scramble" (serves 2)

Spray nonstick skillet with vegetable spray or butter-flavored oil.
Sauté ½ cup minced red pepper and onion and ½ package thawed, drained frozen spinach over low heat until soft.
Add 4 ounces Egg Beaters or 2 whole eggs mixed with 4 egg whites.
Cook at medium heat (eggs should be soft, but not fully scrambled).
Remove from heat and mix in 2 ounces low-fat goat cheese until melted.
Cover pan and return to heat until eggs reach desired doneness.

1 cup strawberries

Wednesday

Fruit and cottage cheese plate

Sprinkle 2 tablespoons chopped nuts on ½ cup low-fat or 2 percent cottage cheese. Surround with 1 cup mixed fruit (berries with chopped apple, chunked melon, fresh peach slices, tangerine, or clementine sections).

Thursday

Mushroom, onion, and ham omelet

Use ½ cup Egg Beaters or egg whites or 1 whole egg mixed with 2 additional egg whites.
A large orange, sectioned, or ½ grapefruit sweetened with Splenda

Friday

Baked apple

Bake with cinnamon and Splenda; sprinkle with 2 tablespoons chopped walnuts.

½ cup vanilla low-fat yogurt

Saturday

Smoked salmon "fingers"

Spread four large endive leaves (or three-inch celery stalks) with low-fat cream cheese. Top each with ½ ounce smoked salmon. Garnish with capers, finely chopped onion, or dill.

½ grapefruit

Sunday

English muffin mound (see selections)

Mound with scrambled eggs, two slices turkey bacon, and one thin slice low-fat Swiss cheese or 3 tablespoons grated low-fat cheddar

1 cup fresh raspberries

Or 1 cup steel-cut oats with ½ cup chopped apples and 2 tablespoons chopped nuts

No cereal, muffins, bagels, toast, or bars except as suggested.

#2—Lunch: Lose the Sandwich and the Pounds Will Follow

In contrast to the changes you need to make at breakfast, this second change should be comparatively painless.

Try a variant on the soup-and-salad theme. This combo makes it easy to fit in those important vegetables and low-fat protein. Any version works:

- Large soup and small salad or veggies from your fridge or the raw bar at the supermarket
- Small soup (as in the 1-cup-size packet) plus a large salad or vegetable entrée

The new lunch is a snap, considering how easy these things are to make and the availability of salads and soups at delis, diners, and fine dining spots. Just figure out where you'll be eating those lunches: home, office, or out. (The car is off-limits here!)

My salad setup is an easy and economical solution for the working woman. Stock up on quart-size take-out containers, and spend about fifteen minutes assembling salad ingredients: greens, raw veggies, and protein (turkey, tuna, shrimp, feta cheese, low-fat cold cuts, hard-boiled eggs) for two to three lunches at a time.

You can even use leftovers from dinner if you make (or buy) a little extra chicken or fish the night before. You put the dressing in first (or carry it separately), then you add the greens, top with raw veggies and protein, and store in the fridge. Shake (gently) five or six times to distribute dressing, and enjoy! You can also do a scoop of tuna or chicken or egg salad (use our fat-reduced recipes, not the ones from the deli) on a big bed of greens and raw vegetables.

Most workplaces have microwaves, so other choices are leftovers from dinner (protein and veggies only), frozen or canned or dry prepackaged meals, and frozen calorie-reduced entrees. (Choose Weight Watchers, Healthy Choice, Amy's, etc.) Round this out with some extra veggies (a small pack of fresh carrots, 1 cup frozen vegetables, or a small salad) and a piece of fruit.

If you are part of the take-out scene at your workplace, there are lots of great options:

- Go with a chef's salad, Greek salad, or chicken Caesar, dressing on the side. Take along your own bottle of low-calorie salad dressing or balsamic vinegar so that you're not at the mercy of the salad maker.
- If you opt for Italian, you can go with an order of broccoli or broccoli rabe ("light on the olive oil") and a small side salad.
- If it's Chinese, stay with the wonton soup (ask them to hold the wontons and add extra strips of chicken and vegetables) or steamed veggies with shrimp or chicken—just remember to order luncheon-size and see whether low-sodium soy or a ponzu-flavored sauce is available.
- Japanese food has lots of choices. Sushi or miso-flavored broths work well.
- For low-calorie Mexican, order chicken or beef fajitas with lots of salsa. Just be sure to forgo the tortilla in any form.

If you are one of the "ladies who lunch" (for whatever reason), the first decision you need to make is where. Check out the "eating-out" strategies in chapter 21. Most restaurants have a large number of choices to accommodate the new breed of diners who are carb modifiers or carb restrictors. Just remember to watch the portion size, or order from the appetizer section of the menu. Good choices are:

- Salads (sans dressing or dressing on the side)
- Egg-white omelets
- Turkey burgers
- Vegetable plates with grilled vegetables or sautéed broccoli (ordered "light on the olive oil")

Eating out is easy if you avoid the bread basket and French fries (or coleslaw) on the side.

#3—Add a Fourth Meal at Four P.M.

The 4 p.m. feeding frenzy is a well-described phenomenon. Years ago, *Vogue* magazine described a beauty salon scenario where during holiday time, platters of goodies put out at 4 p.m. were devoured within minutes by ultrathin clients converging from all corners. Late afternoon is accompanied by increased hunger in all women—the thin, the not-so-thin, the overworked, the overpampered—all get hungry as the day draws to a close. Clearly, it's a universal problem that deserves attention. It doesn't matter whether the cause is fatigue, hunger, stress, hormones, or all of the above.

You need a coping strategy here because a lot of damage can be done in a very short time if it's not part of scheduled eating. Four (or five p.m., depending on when you eat lunch and when you plan to eat dinner) is a good time for a minimeal to thwart overeating at the evening meal. Plan to have a protein and a carb and beverage, and you'll have greater control over caloric consumption and overconsumption later on. This is a great time for:

- A piece of fruit
- A 1-ounce pack of pretzels, or
- A string cheese or 1 ounce of another reduced-fat cheese

Plus

- 8–12 ounces of V8 juice
- A cup of hot spiced tea or Diet Snapple tea

If it's drive time, store an apple or an orange in the car along with a bottled beverage or a nonperishable single-serving cheese (such as Laughing Cow Light).

Unless you're an early-bird dinner person (in which case you can move the fourth meal of the day to 9 p.m.), this needs to be part of your diet arsenal forever.

Wiggle Room

You can see that you have lots of wiggle room with the Carb-Modified Diet. No more need to look for loopholes—places that allow leeway in making those food choices—before you start this diet. The great news is that this type of carb modification doesn't spell deprivation, and you don't have to make drastic changes in your eating to move into this carb-modified mode. Read on for additional details from my workplace to yours.

Chapter 17

THE RIGHT STUFF:
GETTING YOUR KITCHEN IN GEAR

Start with a Shopping Spree

HERE ARE A FEW MORE DETAILS to take the Mogul Protocol to your kitchen and beyond. Start at the supermarket. Even if you are one of the lucky few with someone else in the kitchen (mom, dad, significant other, or offspring), you'll need to have a supply of supplements on hand to keep things under control in case cravings hit. Fresh fruits, frozen low-fat, no-sugar-added ice-cream bars, and low-calorie beverages can be very handy to have around between meals. The number of new options is exploding as manufacturers seek new markets of dieting Americans. Have fun exploring the aisles to restock your shelves. Use the shopping suggestions on pages 102 and 165 for ideas, and be sure that you're not misled by reincarnations of products that sound too good to be true.

If you live anywhere near any of the stores that sell in bulk, like Wal-Mart/Sam's Club, Costco, or BJ's, it will be worth your while to take a trip to stock up on large sizes of many excellent products for healthy eating and bulk cooking at reduced prices. (Try the multiple-serving-size packages of fresh, uncooked, and frozen cooked chicken breasts, Egg Beaters, no-sugar-added ice-cream bars, and vegetables and fruits in quantity.)

If you have a big family and/or a big freezer, you can save time and money. Some memberships even let you shop online for extra convenience. This is an even better way to stay away from store displays of supersized candy, cookies, cakes, and cereals that can only add extra pounds. Online shopping also helps you avoid sampling those 200-calorie-per-bite tidbits they give away as part of the ritual of big-box shopping. Regardless of where you shop, though, watch out for manufacturers' claims of "lowered" carbohydrates based on "net" carbs. The FDA has rejected these terms because they are based on false and faulty advertisements. A carb is a carb is a carb, and "net" carbs make no sense to scientists.

Avoid adulterated, processed, pulverized, and powdered foods with less fiber, higher glycemic loads, and more calories. Stay as fresh as you can.

For the Fridge and Freezer

- Fresh vegetables
- Low-glycemic-index fruits
- Eggs or frozen or egg-white substitutes
- Fresh fish and seafood
- Sliced cooked turkey, chicken breasts, and low-fat ground turkey and chicken
- Low-fat sliced deli meats and low-fat hot dogs that have no more than fifty calories (turkey dogs are good)
- Low-fat turkey or tofu sausage and turkey bacon
- Frozen veggie combos without sauce or pasta
- Frozen veggie burgers and vegetable patties
- Canned and frozen soups with fewer than 120 calories per 1-cup serving
- Frozen low-fat ice-cream bars (4-ounce and a maximum of 120 calories per serving) and no-sugar-added, low-fat ice cream
- Plain yogurt (or 6- to 8-ounce containers of low-fat yogurt with Splenda or Equal)
- Low-fat cheeses (bulk, sliced, or shredded)

To Stock Your Shelves

- Olive oil spray
- Splenda granulated and packets; Equal packets and boxes
- Canned vegetable or low-sodium chicken stock (or cubes or powdered versions)

- Balsamic vinegar
- Mustards in all flavors as long as they have fewer than thirty calories per tablespoon (watch out for honey mustards)
- Low-carb ketchup (regular ketchup is high in sugar)
- Canned tomatoes and tomato sauce with fewer than sixty calories per ½-cup serving
- Jars of salsa, Chinese sauces, Japanese sauces, miso, horseradish sauce, chunky vegetable mixtures (tapenade, caponata, bruschetta) that are thirty calories or fewer per tablespoon (avoid barbecue sauces), peppers
- Sun-dried tomatoes (dry ones only)
- Canned tuna, shrimp, sardines
- Teas, all flavors, all varieties
- Bottles of diet or unsweetened iced tea, water, diet soda

Current Kudos

Let's get specific. Here's my latest list from the latest low-cal entries at the supermarket (plus just a few favorites that have stood the test of time). I use these in my own kitchen because I think they please the palate *and* prime the scale. Many have that unbeatable combo of low fat and no sugar and contain real ingredients. I try these out side by side with their higher-calorie cousins to make sure they are tasty as well as healthy. Otherwise, why bother?

- Heinz One Carb Reduced Sugar Ketchup: Five calories per tablespoon and 1 gram of carbohydrates. This is a truly fantastic condiment, indistinguishable from the original.
- Hellman's light or Kraft low-calorie olive oil mayonnaise: These are as good as it gets for reduced-calorie mayo.
- College Inn Vegetable Stock: This twenty-five-calorie-a-cup soup is a great pick-me-up as is and a fantastic base for all manner of homemade soups and sauces.
- Ken's Steakhouse light olive oil and balsamic vinegar and Caesar dressings: These have been around for a while, but they always make my list. They are my gold standards. You can decalorize these further by pouring off the oil in the bottle and replacing it with vegetable stock, wine, or apple cider.
- Aunt Gussie's low-fat, sugar-free garlic flat crackers (www.auntgussies.com): These large (six-inch oval) crackers

are only forty-five calories each, contain all natural ingredients, and taste crunchy and buttery.

- Smart Balance light margarine in a tub: It has no trans fats, is lactose free, and works well in vegetarian and kosher kitchens.
- Starbucks no-sugar-added brownie: Here's a way to get portion control for that weekly treat. This three-inch-square goodie has the flavor of real bittersweet chocolate without an overly sweet or chemical taste that's found in other low-fat brownies on the market.
- Trader Joe's red pepper caponata: See Trader Joe's website (www. traderjoes.com) for a wide range of reduced-calorie and natural products that make it easy to stay on track at a surprisingly low cost. Their caponatas can be used as dips or spreads or sauces right from the jar, or they can be combined with mayo for an astonishingly easy-to-make and flavorful accompaniment to grilled fish or chicken. You can add three or four tablespoons to an equal volume of coarsely chopped, cooked vegetables (onions, mushrooms, zucchini) to top pasta or use them to thicken juice from the roast for a great gravy.
- Progresso chicken or turkey soups: At 90–100 calories a cup and 180–200 calories a can, these soups deliver a flavorful and filling alternative to lots of other fast foods. With new flip-top lids, they are easily transportable and can turn any office with a microwave into an almost effortless source for lunch in minutes.

The Well-Equipped Kitchen

You want a kitchen that's well equipped with the proper pans and tools to simplify food preparation. Twelve kitchen aids to decalorize foods include the following:

- **Large, good-quality, nonstick sauté pan, frying pan, or a wok with a cover.**
  This is essential for stir-frying and sautéing. Nonstick coatings can now be heated to much higher temperatures, with just the barest trace of oil, so you can sear and lock in flavor when cooking vegetables and meats, eliminating hundreds of extra calories. (Use some vegetable cooking spray or wipe a single tablespoon of oil on the pan surface with a paper towel.) Go with a pan made of

stainless steel or a combination of sturdy metals. There are many excellent choices in a range of prices, and some of the lowest-priced pans work just as well as the most expensive ones.

- **Eight- to twelve-quart stockpot**
  When you're on the Carb-Modified Diet, you'll find that soup is a mainstay—a healthy alternative to sandwiches at lunch and starches at dinner. So you must have a soup pot to make satisfying soups that decrease appetite and are usually healthy, unless you add lots of butter, cream, or fatty meats to the pot. Soups are inexpensive meals, and you can make large quantities of an endless variety of great soups in a short time. (By the way, the soup-making formula on page 176 makes every one of us a virtual chef!)

- **Measuring spoons**
  You need spoons for measuring oils, mayonnaise, salad dressings, sauces, and condiments that are more than thirty calories per tablespoon.

- **Ice-cream scoop (½-cup size)**
  Ice-cream scoops can be used for lots more than ice cream. Use them to measure starches (rice, mashed potatoes) and to calibrate the correct serving size of salads (tuna, chicken, shrimp) that you can scoop onto greens at lunch. Stay with the smaller ⅓- to ½-cup size (not the jumbo scoop) to make sure you don't accidentally measure out a cup or more.

- **Kitchen scale calibrated in half-ounces or grams**
  This is how you learn to eyeball portion sizes so that you won't overdose on cheese, meats, nuts, and other healthy but caloric foods that you must eat in limited quantities to lose weight.

- **Glass measuring cup**
  If you're buying only one, get a 2-cup size. Use this as a visual guide to approximate the correct portion size of a pasta serving. (You will not need it to measure most other foods on this program.)

- **Plastic containers and storage/freezer plastic bags**
  You need a variety of containers and bags for storing, freezing, and transporting food. Disposable and reusable plastic containers help you control your portions. Also, save the plastic containers you get with deli foods. Fill the 1-quart size with individual-size salads or the 1-pint size with soup or leftovers

for lunch at work. Plastic storage bags make it easy to add cut-up carrots and other veggies to lunch boxes. They are also useful for storing leftover servings of meat, fish, seafood, cheese, fresh herbs, and other sauce-free scraps to add to future meals. Larger bags suitable for freezing are a good way to extend the season of those wonderful berries at peak flavor and low price from the all-too-short months of summer.

- **Wire or mesh strainer**
  Use a strainer to drain and rinse unwanted sauces from otherwise healthy foods. This helps you easily decalorize foods made in your own kitchen and in those of others. Drain salad dressings from deli salads. Remove countless excess calories and extra salt from canned fish (tuna, anchovies, sardines) and prepared vegetables marinated or cooked in oil. You can use warm water for degreasing most of these and boiling water to remove oil and bring grilled (and other) vegetables from the deli counter to room temperature without removing flavor. This is my favorite way to expand options for healthy takeout and put vegetables on the plate in seconds.

- **Kitchen shears**
  These are invaluable for "bite sizing." Convert slices of deli meats and low-fat cheeses to strips for use in a chef's salad. And create chunks of shrimp, sausage, hot dogs, or cooked chicken breast for other combos. Your shears can mince fresh herbs (parsley, chives), sun-dried tomatoes, anchovies—lots of things you can use to dress up foods and enhance presentation. They are also handy for opening blister packs, removing skin from meats, and deboning chicken breasts.

- **Stand-up shredder/grater**
  It's amazing how much flavor you can add to food with one-half ounce of shredded low-fat cheddar (or jalapeño jack cheese) or freshly grated parmesan cheese per serving (two ounces for four servings). These are great last-minute additions to many egg dishes (scrambles, omelets, frittatas) and a wonderful topping for baked potatoes, chili, casseroles, and soups. Shredded cheese melts easily and enhances visual appeal as well as taste without adding a lot of calories. Grated cheese is de rigueur for many pasta dishes and can be mixed into bread crumbs as a coating for fish or chicken. If your family likes

these dishes, shred some cheddar in advance and store it in a plastic storage bag.

- **Small electric food chopper or a good chef's knife**
These choppers make it easy to have minced onions, peppers, mushrooms, and parsley on hand to add to omelets and other healthy dishes. If you're a budding (or seasoned) chef, you may enjoy emulating Emeril and using a chef's knife to chop herbs, nuts, garlic, shallots, onions, and other essential ingredients, as time and inclination permit.

- **Blender, food processor, or immersion blender**
This is an excellent investment in weight management. Soups are so easy to make—just fifteen to thirty minutes in the kitchen can produce many quarts of soup for your fridge and freezer. Even if you like chunky soups, the flavor will be much more intense if you puree part of the liquid and mix this into the rest of the pot. Buy a hand-held "immersion" blender to do this without the mess of getting the stockpot contents into the food processor. One additional caveat: you can avoid burning your hands and ruining countertops by simply letting the contents cool before you use these devices.

Chapter 18

YOU CAN'T BE TOO ORGANIZED

Making It Easy to Turn Out Healthy Food

NOW YOU GET TO REAP THE BENEFITS of all your preparations. You've filled your prescription, cleaned out your cupboards, restocked your shelves, and you're ready to get your act together in the kitchen.

For someone with Syndrome W, this is truly a new era in your weight-loss history. Finally, you have a medication to address the underlying metabolic defect that's responsible for your midlife weight gain and waist expansion, along with a diet grounded in science, not promises! All you need now is a bit of planning and kitchen preparation to maximize success. Here's a set of strategies to feed you and others at your table and leave time for other important activities for you as well as all those significant others in your life.

Modular Meals

Modular meal planning is an effective way to produce tasty, nutritious meals with a minimum of last-minute fuss and cleanup. I used this strategy for many years when I was a working woman with three children and a heavy round of carpooling and errands every afternoon. The last thing I needed to face at the end of the day was the hassle of cooking from scratch. But I also thought that eating out, even for a woman who's better known for making restaurant reservations than making meals, is somewhat disappointing on a steady basis (it's expensive, often fattening, and eventually boring). I never thought that picking up take-out food worked much better because healthy, tasty, and reasonably priced alternatives to the eat-in emporiums in the malls of Main Street America were also hard to find.

That's what motivated me to come up with my modular meals. This game plan required two Sunday mornings a month, when I cooked to stock the freezer with family-size portions of family favorites. These included turkey chili, chicken casseroles, vegetable lasagna, meatloaf, meatballs, and hearty stews. I even baked a bunch of russet potatoes, scooped out the contents, and flavored the mix with chives, cottage cheese, buttermilk—anything but butter—and wrapped the potatoes individually in foil wrap. I'd make large batches of rice, pasta, and bulgur wheat; use some in my casseroles; and store the rest separately for the starch part of the equation (see the recipes in part V).

That was then and this is now. Today, my children are grown, and I no longer carpool, but I'm as busy as ever, so I still use the modular strategy. The only difference is that today, I'm more likely to buy some of my modules because I live in a community that has a wonderful bounty of healthy vegetable takeout. But I still bake potatoes and make little packets of pasta to stack in the freezer (see instructions below), I store the extra brown rice that I take home from my favorite Chinese restaurant, and I always keep a few family-size casseroles in my freezer. That way, when my kids and now grandkids come home, I can save those precious moments we spend together for fun rather than food preparation.

I see variations on this theme in newspapers and magazines (*Real Simple, Cooking Light, Food and Wine, Cook's Illustrated*) and cookbooks. These approaches truly do reduce time, cost, and frenzy.

You'll find lots of great recipes in publications, but do keep in mind that "healthy" doesn't always mean low calorie, and never use the ¼ to ½ cup olive oil that's a standard of American cookbooks. Instead, cut it to ⅛ cup (that's 2 tablespoons or 1 liquid ounce).

Here's the simple equation and an overview of my cooking modules to help your transition to healthy eating. (See recipes and meal plans in part V.)

Dinner = entrée + starch + two vegetables + dessert
(group A) (group B) (group C)

Entrée First

Use either of the two suggestions that follow to avoid overeating simply because there's "nothing good" in the house and dinner has to be on the table in twenty minutes. This eliminates that scenario common to women who get home late and end up eating whatever's easiest, like pizza or other highly caloric takeout. Eat better and simplify your life in the kitchen with one of the following:

1. Combine a main-course fish or meat entrée with some leftovers or (healthy) takeout that you prepare creatively.

or

2. Make it potluck size. Cook in bulk. Make dishes to feed eight to twelve as a main course or a side dish.

Roast a large bone-in or boned turkey breast or a dozen chicken breasts, or bake a large fillet (salmon, bass, snapper) for the first night, and you get lots of options for additional meals. If you're too busy or too tired to cook, find a local deli or supermarket and buy two barbecued chickens or special-order a turkey or turkey breast for a few extra pennies per pound. (Remove the skin before serving.) Fish stores, gourmet shops, and most fish counters at supermarkets will poach a small salmon for you if you ask.

Many recipes lend themselves to supersizing. You'll find very little extra work and no additional cleanup time when you double, triple, and quadruple family favorites. If possible, never cook for one or two! Most dishes can be recycled or reheated for another meal.

Our potluck recipes already include calculations for eight servings to make the math easy. Freeze in one- to four-portion-size plastic containers or microwavable or oven-ready disposable foil pans.

Great choices are turkey chili, fish and seafood stews and chowders, turkey meatloaf, turkey meatballs, and chicken breasts, which can be made in infinite variations, depending on the sauce.

Starch Next

You can precook and package rice, other grains, and pasta for easy access and assembly at mealtime. Make these in bulk as well—two packages of pasta or rice and grain mixtures (omit the recommended oil) or eight servings of plain, preferably whole-grain, or brown rice, wild rice, barley, or quinoa—and freeze in single- or multiple-serving-size plastic bags or plastic containers.

Freeze spaghetti and linguini unadorned or in a small amount of sauce or broth. Penne and other larger tubular pastas are best with at least a light coating of sauce. Cook these al dente (slightly underdone), and they reheat well directly out of the freezer or in additional broth or sauce. One of my oldest strategies is to cook a pound of pasta, and using a measuring cup, store it in single-size plastic bags that I stack in the freezer.

Tips on buying/using freezer bags:

- Use freezer-friendly plastic bags.
- Make sure you select the right size.
- Press out all the air, and flatten them to avoid freezer burn.

Vegetables in the Mix

Although fresh is best, you may not have time to cut, steam, or stir-fry the vegetables and greens that you're adding to your diet. A favorite time-saver for singles and small households is to go to salad bars and buy precut broccoli, cauliflower, mushrooms, and peppers. This can be an expensive option for larger families. But you can also try the handy bags of precut lettuce, broccoli, carrots, and so on available at most grocery stores today.

Fortunately, you can find a great array of frozen vegetables that make excellent side dishes and are also good for stretching the volume and fiber content of foods with sauces. My favorites for fast preparation are broccoli florets, asparagus tips, peas, baby whole string beans, and artichokes. I also like many veggie mixtures. They add variety and a range of vitamins and color to your dinner plate. (Just avoid vegetables with sauces.)

Have two servings of vegetables and a salad at dinner. That's the absolute minimum. Truly, in this case, if a little is good, more is better.

Work the Assembly Line

Now it's time to get dinner on the table. Mix and match by taking one from group A (entrée) and one from group B (the starch) and two from group C (vegetables). Combine a home-cooked entrée with vegetables from the deli counter, or bring in some turkey meatballs from the pizza parlor to top your frozen rice and beans.

Plot your course in advance by calculating your time available and who'll be there to help with meal prep. You might even enlist some help from the troops. Plan ahead; defrost your entrée in the refrigerator overnight unless you have the forty-five minutes to pop the foil pans directly into the oven from the freezer the minute you walk in the door. (Don't leave that casserole on your countertop because you can cause food poisoning if you defrost food for more than two hours at room temperature.) Do whatever works. Family meals can be hectic, but with a little foresight, they can be healthy and happy as well.

Decalorize to Downsize

You can find many easy ways to decalorize food and still retain flavor. Fat and sugar, those calorically dense non-nutrients, add very little to the pleasure of eating. You've probably acquired a few cooking skills by this point in your life. Like the two professional chefs I treated who lost a total of two hundred pounds, you need to use all these skills to help you and your family get healthy and stay that way. Eliminating hidden calories lets you cook and enjoy new and heirloom recipes, once you learn to decalorize.

Some Suggestions to Cut Calories from Favorite Dishes

- Substitute 1–2 tablespoons of olive oil or a herb- or citrus-seasoned vegetable oil to replace the larger quantities of fat in recipes for soups, sauces, stews, and starches. You add flavor without a great cost in calories.
- Stock up on Splenda Granulated, a sugar substitute that measures cup for cup like sugar. Use in cooking and baking to decrease caloric content dramatically. Use it to sweeten baked fruit (peach, blueberry, plum) or pureed fruit (apple, strawberry, pear).
- Puree vegetables to thicken the sauce that binds with greater nutritional value than traditional thickeners like butter mixed with flour or cornstarch.
- Bake traditional "fried foods" like chicken cutlets, fish, or eggplant slices in a crust coating to minimize fat content without sacrificing flavor.
- Roast your "sautéed" dishes (hash browns and other potatoes) with 1–2 tablespoons of olive oil or flavored oil and a sprinkling

of dry seasoning, onion soup, or salad dressing. This makes a tasty, easy-to-prepare side dish.

- Steam vegetables and vegetable combos; then add any of the following for four (one-cup) servings:

  - 1–2 tablespoons of a "light" margarine made without trans fats (Smart Balance is excellent and works well in kosher kitchens)
  - 1 tablespoon sesame oil or ½ tablespoon hot pepper oil plus 1 tablespoon another vegetable oil

Use the Two-Cup Pasta Rule

I've never met a patient who didn't rank pasta as the dish she *most* missed on restrictive low-carb diets she tried and abandoned. You don't have to be Italian to love lasagna (and spaghetti and tortellini and cavatelli). But you do have to learn what constitutes a serving and understand that it's not the average plateful that many Americans eat as an individual serving in a single sitting. Clearly, our penchant for pasta knows no bounds. In the United States, restaurants typically serve you pasta in two- to three-cup portions. Even a half-portion appetizer is a cup or more. So, in the words of Shakespeare, "There's the rub."

You can find a way to integrate pasta into your Carb-Modified Diet because pasta is not off-limits. You can use my simple way to incorporate pasta—the real thing, not the ersatz protein-based product—into a dinner (only) that totally conforms to your new eating plan. You just revise the ratio of sauce to substance.

The traditional view of pasta calls for one-half cup of sauce to one cup-plus of pasta, as in pasta with marinara, Bolognese, pesto, amatriciana, puttanesca—you name it. So, you simply rewrite this ratio and change your concept of the sauce component.

Instead of tomatoes, oil, cream, cheese, or any combo thereof, think vegetables, fish, seafood, chicken, and turkey. You have an infinite number of combinations and permutations to choose from with pasta; you can use mushrooms, onions, peppers (red, green, yellow, orange), broccoli, broccoli rabe, eggplant, artichoke hearts, zucchini, shrimp, scallops, salmon, tuna (fresh or canned), chicken cubes, turkey strips, and on and on.

This is an opportunity for culinary creativity. **Just stick to the two-cup rule:**

- Two cups of sauce to one cup of pasta if this is the main component of dinner, or
- One cup of sauce to one-half cup of pasta if it's a side dish

This strategy also translates to restaurant eating and takeout. You can find pasta with broccoli, broccoli rabe, and seafood in both low-end and upscale establishments. Restaurant owners are becoming increasingly responsive to the needs of weight-conscious diners, and the ones who aren't may wind up seeing their places crossed off your list. Most chefs devote their talents to sauces, so that means they usually won't be offended if you ask them to downsize your pasta.

To correct what my psychiatrist daughter calls "cognitive food distortions," haul out your measuring cup (glass) to reprogram your portion perceptions. You have to learn what a single cup of pasta looks like on a plate or in a shallow bowl. (It's about the size of an average clenched fist.)

Add your two-cup combo of vegetable, chicken, or fish "sauce" and even another half-cup of bite-size green vegetables (peas, broccoli florets, asparagus tips) if you want more volume. Take an extra minute or two to serve pasta in individual servings; never, ever serve it family style because then you won't be able to gauge how much you're eating.

Sit down and enjoy your pasta dish guilt free, knowing that you're operating within the confines of your Carb-Modified Diet. You may even find, with this revised ratio, that you have leftover sauce to use with vegetables for tomorrow's lunch.

Go Crustless

At a restaurant or a friend's dinner party, you can eliminate crust (on "crusted" foods) by scraping it off or working around it—and thus save numerous high-fat calories. The flavor is typically in the filling, so you're much better off eating the apples from the apple pie, the veggies from the spring roll, or the spinach from the knish.

When you cook at home, you can eliminate crusts, too. You can transform pumpkin pie, quiche, and cheesecake (as your weekly treat) by spraying a light coating of vegetable oil in a soufflé dish and then cooking the filling "nude" in a bain-marie (a second pan filled two-thirds with water) in a 350°F oven (or you can dust the soufflé dish with a few bread or graham cracker crumbs before you pour in the filling).

By the way, rolling fish in seasoned crumbs for a crust makes an excellent entrée. (See recipes in part V.)

Use Generic

Generics work in the kitchen as well as the pharmacy. I often use my prescription pad to diagram pictures of generic recipes that work for weight loss. My favorites are my generic soups, salad, and pasta combo. I believe that a few basic recipes are the key to overcoming overweight long-term. Each of these has numerous variations. All you have to do is tailor them to your tastes and the vegetables of the season and the hues that make you happy. See the recipe section for green and orange soups, my salad "shaker," and pasta plates.

Now that you've reorganized your kitchen and revamped your cooking style, you're totally on course.

Part IV

YOUR LIFESTYLE:
Strategies for Change

This section helps you identify and overcome barriers to weight loss and integrate eating behaviors that maximize your likelihood of overcoming weight gain long-term. You discover how easy it is to stay on track with the Mogul Protocol everywhere you go. And, once you have all the key information under your belt, you'll see that your only future concern with weight will be that lovely one called "maintenance."

I also share my somewhat unique perspective on the merits and myths of exercise in women. My finale includes a few new handouts and FAQs from a decade of dialogues. Here are all the rules and tools and insights that will help you to create your own manual for weight loss . . . forever.

Chapter 19

FACTS AND FIGURES:
LOSING WEIGHT BY GETTING SCIENCE

A Few Good Books and Many Groundbreaking Studies

MOST OF US HAVE A FEW DIET BOOKS on our shelves. Each promises all-new insights, miracle cures, and ways to eat everything we would like to eat yet stay "forever thin."

The first few chapters follow a formula: a physician, psychologist, celebrity, or the common man talks about his or her discovery, that unwanted byproduct of maturity—the mature body during its transition into adulthood. After soul-searching and unsuccessful attempts to reverse the contour changes and the weight gain and overcome the aging process, the writer finally finds the Holy Grail on the road to becoming the next diet guru. Each epiphany for altering the energy equation generates the next best-selling diet book for the ever-expanding audience of readers who are always seeking that elusive quick fix.

With a few notable exceptions, such tomes generically promise rapid weight loss by means of simple solutions based on pseudoscience. They don't bother to take into account the great progress that has been made in the evolving science of obesity.

A few books even refer to some of the well-conducted studies that actually can facilitate weight loss for the 45 percent of women and the 30 percent of American men who are always "on a diet." The explosion of scientific research in response to the alarming escalation of the national obesity epidemic has taught us a lot about what works and what doesn't.

Neuroscientists have deconstructed the black box of "appetite" and "satiety." State-of-the-art studies of eating behaviors in million-dollar clinical research centers in New York, New Orleans, Boston, and Houston, and clinical trials in Atlanta and San Antonio have all provided fascinating new insights into the relationship between food intake and fat storage, cell signals and cellulite formation, and the importance of food quality and timing in weight management. Snippets from ground-breaking studies air on the evening news and dot the pages of the *New York Times*, the *Wall Street Journal*, and *USA Today*.

This body of research is a treasure trove that provides support for the treatment methods our team has used and studied for the past three decades—explanations from other laboratories and other populations that show why the things we propose and use do work. These findings represent the scientific advancements of hundreds of committed research scientists. As summarized by Tara Parker-Pope in the *Wall Street Journal*, November 2003, "The diet that works isn't based on a single big idea. Instead, it's a set of scientifically based tools that are essential to weight loss."

Cracking the obesity code has been a formidable task for many talented researchers. How exciting to look at their collective findings to support "proof of concept" for our dietary program and our protocol! Best of all, what we've learned through extensive research and experience can help you lose weight and regain your figure. Knowledge is power!

Facts, Not Fancy

Conspicuous Consumption

Fact #1: Calories do count.

When I was growing up, the bestseller *Calories Don't Count* hit the charts. The first of a long list of such books, this one challenged old teachings about the energy equation, selling a new message based on new scientific evidence. It pitched the idea that caloric balance was outmoded, ill conceived, and unimportant to lifetime weight regulation. Unfortunately, this fallacy was picked up and carried on, a banner that became the underpinning of many diets devised since the 1960s.

Apparently, the concept of caloric balance is just not sexy. The notion that weight gain results from too many calories consumed for the number of calories expended doesn't turn people on or sell books. It's true but boring.

Countless diet-book authors have challenged the concept of caloric balance and offered "replacement theories" that were supposedly based on good science. *But the proof is in the fattening pudding.* Obesity in Americans of all ages and ethnicities has continued to spiral upward. Sadly, all effective diets—high-protein, high-carbohydrate, low-fat, low-sugar, grapefruit diet, ice-cream diet—work only because they ultimately reduce caloric intake. Any plan that doesn't lead to lowered calories just doesn't produce meaningful loss of weight and excess body fat.

We all love novelty and simple solutions. The past few decades have promised immediate weight loss if you'll just:

- Gorge on bacon and eggs
- Curtail your carbohydrates
- Consume excessive amounts of fruits (as long as other foods are eliminated)
- Restrict all sugar or just white sugar and white carbs

Such diets inspire confidence, easily draw converts, and may even deliver short-term weight loss. Unfortunately, expert after expert always come to one conclusion—that the real news on diet is depressing. The most successful diets, even with intense medical supervision, lead to early weight loss in the first six months, followed by a plateau of six months, and finally, regain of weight.

In fact, long-term weight reduction is so unusual that the National Institutes of Health created a registry so that those few lucky individuals who figure out how to lose weight and keep it off for two or more years could share their secrets with the scientists responsible for public health recommendations about diet and exercise!

Long-term weight loss is indeed rare, and that's because it happens only when a dietary regimen (or exercise program) produces *a net caloric deficit* over time. A calorie is a calorie is a calorie, and 3,500 calories will always equal a pound. Overconsumption of as little as 10 calories (one potato chip) a day will produce a weight gain of one pound a year, or ten pounds per decade. Reduce your daily intake by 150 calories a day (one can of soda), and you'll lose fifteen pounds in a year.

A rigorous study of patients who followed a popular carb-restricted regimen for six months showed that study subjects lost weight by cutting carbs simply because they ate less overall. When they limited their carbohydrates and other foods that were allowed, they consumed fewer calories. It's what nutritionists call the "no crackers, less cheese" rule.

As an endocrinologist, I've had a unique opportunity to evaluate and treat hormonal conditions that cause weight gain or decrease weight loss in motivated women despite good efforts in regard to diet and exercise. No question, subtle (and not-so-subtle) endocrine disturbances can make weight management difficult. Thyroid problems, cortisol excess, growth hormone deficiency (seen in patients with pituitary tumors and other pituitary abnormalities), and undetected insulin elevations all make it hard for people to shed excess pounds. Correcting these endocrine defects, typically with hormone replacement or other treatments, facilitates but never guarantees weight loss. *You still have to diet and/or exercise regularly. Long-term weight loss requires lifestyle changes and ongoing dietary vigilance.* Any physician, nutritional counselor, diet guru, or author who promises otherwise is ill informed and irresponsible and not really telling the truth!

Finding Syndrome W is all about uncovering a commonly missed metabolic defect that blunts weight-loss efforts in formerly thin or average-size midlife women. But treating Syndrome W still requires dietary change. Metformin is not magic. It enables, but does not eliminate, the caloric restriction necessary to lose weight. The energy equation still reigns supreme. Calories do count.

There's No Free Lunch (Breakfast, Dinner, or Snack)

Fact #2: Fiber and fluid make you full.

One of the hottest areas of obesity study is the new science of appetite regulation. Market-driven research and the potential windfall of "curing" or controlling obesity have spawned a new look at the old question, "How do we get obese American adults and children to stop eating so much?"

We eat early; we eat often. Our lives center on food, and Big Gulps and Double Whoppers have programmed us to eat quantities of food so large they could have fed an entire family a generation ago.

We understand that it's a matter of portion size. But when restaurants serve three cups of pasta as a standard-size serving, it's hard to be happy with the one-half cup that the nutrition community calls a proper carb serving.

Dieting puts us out of sync with America's fast- (and not-so-fast) food eateries and big-box stores. "Less is more" also conflicts with the basic survival skills of our ancestors, who scavenged and stored energy sources. Plus, it also goes against bargain-hunting behaviors embedded in our brains when we're in early childhood.

Truthfully, you have only two ways to cut calories and live in the real world of food:

- Decrease the caloric density (the number of calories per gram) of the foods you eat
- Learn to be satisfied with less food

Nothing else gives you the caloric dip you need in order to lose weight.

What's the least painful route that's still effective? Choose foods with a low caloric density and make them the base of your diet. This means eating lots more of the following:

- Vegetables
- High-fiber fruits
- Low-fat protein
- Low-fat dairy products

You may take some detours along the way, but you'll discover there's no other true path to long-term weight control.

Many studies have shown that diets high in vegetables, fruit, and fiber lead to long-term weight loss. New studies are unearthing facts that explain exactly why this is true. The old-fashioned idea of eating fruits and vegetables for weight loss has a very new-fashioned scientific foundation: the effect of "gut peptides" on brain chemistry.

Sixties-era researchers started exploring the physiology of food intake. Early on, after charting the eating behaviors of laboratory animals (mice, rats, guinea pigs, rabbits), scientists observed that most animals didn't eat continuously even when given access to food day and night. Somewhere, somehow, built-in mechanisms made them stop eating. It appeared that certain nerve impulses or cell substances served as a mind-meal connection to halt feeding. The researchers proposed that satiety signals from the gut could be regulating meal size.

Fast-forward to the twenty-first century, and you see the picture is almost complete after the identification and isolation of hormones that control short-term food intake and long-term weight regulation. You perceive fullness based on the volume and content of what you eat.

Two important regulators with opposite effects appear to be key players in the circuitry. One from the stomach—ghrelin—turns on eating; a second—PYY—from the duodenum, turns it off. Sophisticated studies are now under way, looking for answers as to how and why the brain perceives different foods differently. Eating large volumes of food of low caloric density will reduce your appetite, and we are beginning to understand how!

Ghrelin and Girth

Fact #3: Hunger is all in your head.

Ghrelin is the hot new hunger hormone. After you eat a meal, ghrelin goes down, but it rises steadily over the next few hours until it reaches a critical level and tells your brain, "Time to eat another meal." You reach the highest ghrelin level at 2 a.m., which may account for night eating in those of you who stay up late.

Several factors regulate ghrelin production. One is the volume of food in your stomach because the decline in ghrelin is what signals fullness and tells you it's time to stop, put down your fork, and leave the table.

According to several studies, bariatric surgery that reduces the size of the stomach also reduces ghrelin levels. This is an important mechanism that leads to decreased food intake and weight loss after gastric bypass surgery. Ghrelin has also been given part of the blame for the new association of sleep deprivation with appetite excess. Ghrelin levels rise when sleep declines below four hours per night, and the food preferences of those sleep-deprived subjects were all in the high-carb categories (candies, cookies, cakes, and pretzels).

Fluids and foods influence ghrelin differently. Plain water doesn't reduce ghrelin, but water with added sugar or salt produces a significant change. This suggests that your brain perceives water differently from the way it perceives food. These studies fit with studies of fullness in humans, like the one at Penn State that showed women who ate chicken rice soup lost more weight than women who had the identical meal but ate it as eight ounces of water plus chicken rice casserole. The book *Volumetrics*, by Dr. Barbara Rolls, summarizes this research.

The Mogul Protocol's Carb-Modified Diet is high in vegetables, low-fat proteins, and "acceptable" fruit and fiber. These dietary recommendations have worked well for more than a generation of women I've treated in three decades of medical practice. What's different today is the metformin we've added to complete the picture and make it far easier for

women to take off weight. Our data and those of other researe
that metformin lowers the levels of ghrelin in the bloodstream.

Getting the Glycemic Index and the Glycemic Load

Fact #4: Let glycemic load lead the way.

Glycemic Index (GI) is a measure of the similarity of a given food to
sugar, which has a glycemic index of 1.0. Search the term on the Internet (with Google or another search engine), and you'll find a number
of websites that list glycemic indexes of common foods. The higher
the glycemic index, the more a food acts like sugar, raising your blood
sugar and stimulating insulin production.

If you're a diabetic, using the GI to modify your diet can decrease
spikes in your blood sugar and improve long-term glucose control. If
you have Syndrome W or an abnormal insulin response curve, it can
also smooth out the ups and downs of your insulin production throughout the day. When you factor in the serving size of the carbohydrate,
you have what's called the glycemic load.

The GI is tricky because it's based on measurements of a single food,
and we usually eat mixtures. One meal may include carbohydrates, protein, and fat. Therefore, the GI of the carbs you eat is a great guide, but
it doesn't tell the whole story. How high your sugar rises when you eat
a cookie or a carrot doesn't depend on only the GI of these items. It
depends on the fat content of the cookie and how much protein and
other fiber you eat along with the carrot. Understanding the principles
of the GI is very helpful and lets you subdivide fruits and grains into
low- and high-glycemic-index categories. My patients find this a lot
easier than fixating on the GI of every food.

In simplest terms, the more fiber and the higher the water content
of a fruit or grain product, the lower the glycemic index. That's why you
should strictly limit dried fruits and fruit juices. Eat grapes rather than
raisins. Choose an orange over canned (unsweetened) orange segments and unsweetened orange juice. By the same token, whole oats
with intact fiber are better than instant oats, and brown rice is better
than white rice.

Get in the habit of eating low-GI fruits (citrus fruits and berries)
and whole-grain fiber-rich carbs as part of the long-term dietary
changes you'll need to make for lower weight and better health.

In recent years, key GI concepts have sometimes been distorted
beyond good sense. Some people point to the GI to justify choosing

ıked potato (the fat in the fries lowers the GI) or
ɔ for abandoning healthy foods like carrots (with a
packaged products with lower nutrient value (based
ıtent of vitamins and flavonoids).

marily for comparing fruits, vegetables, and starches
ʃdrates). Don't use it as license to overdose on candies
n increasing array of packaged products and mixes for
ca.   ., and pancakes that claim to have a low glycemic index.

Read the e labels carefully. The new exclusion of alcohol "sugars" in calculating GI is just old deceptive advertising. It's reminiscent of the way people embraced low-fat Oreos a decade ago.

The GI is a great guide to healthy eating, but remember to interpret it sensibly. *Caveat emptor!*

The Lowdown on Low Carbs

Fact #5: Low-carb diets cut calories.

Finally, after Americans converted to low-carb lifestyles, as sales of Krispy Kremes plummeted and sugar-free Snackwells skyrocketed, results from several low-carb-diet clinical trials began to emerge. Three studies in 2003 challenged traditional views of the optimal balance of carbs, fat, and protein for weight loss.

Nutrition experts responded by citing these conclusions:

- Ad-lib high-fat diets worked because they limited food choices.
- These diets produced weight loss comparable to and possibly better than traditional, high-carb diets in the short term (six months).
- One-year weight loss was poor with both dietary extremes.

My view is that the high-fat (low-carb) diet of the 1970s is *not* the answer to the high-carb (low-fat) diet of the 1990s. The 2003 dietary studies demonstrate the low success rates of restrictive diets in general and reinforce the virtues of a regimen that provides a wide variety of food choices and avoids all calorically dense foods, whether fats, simple sugars, carbohydrates, or protein.

Timing Is Everything

Fact #6: When you eat is as important as what you eat.

A landmark study from the Clinical Research Center at Harvard (published in 1999) showed that the glycemic indexes of the foods you eat for breakfast determine how much you eat later in the day. This study of overweight, nondiabetic adolescents underscored that a low-glycemic-index breakfast not only has a beneficial effect on the production of important fuels in the body, as well as stress hormones, appetite signals, and neurotransmitters for the following four hours, but decreases food intake many hours later. Thus, you can see the advantages of eating your starches later in the day, a recommendation that is the cornerstone of our Carb-Modified Diet.

Making Sense of Macronutrients

Fact #7: Low-fat and low-carb diets make you fat when you freeload.

Nutritionists like to talk about macronutrients, carbohydrates, fats, and proteins. How should these be balanced to promote weight loss? How about their role in overall health? We see opinions in hundreds of scientific papers, magazine articles, research studies, news commentaries, and celebrity talk shows. You can even get friendly advice from the man on the street. Dietary evangelism greets us everywhere we go in America.

To lose weight, should we cut carbs or fat? This great diet debate probably won't be resolved anytime soon, but strong evidence exists that high-fat diets promote heart disease and many types of cancer. But there's no consensus about the converse.

As stated on page 1 in the *New York Times* (October 2004) report on congressional hearings evaluating Medicare reimbursement for the medical management of obesity: "At the current time there is no available data to demonstrate that any current weight-reduction regimen is effective either for long-term weight maintenance or for any other meaningful health outcome measure." More recently (January 2005), a study of the ten most popular diets used by Americans provided little evidence that any of the regimens worked.

To lose weight, avoid foods high in density of fat *or* sugar *or* protein (like compressed protein bars), and all diet delights that deliver a large number of calories per gram. Foods that contain two of these—fat, sugar, and protein—in one bite (cookies, cakes, candies, and many cereals) need to get off your shopping list forever.

You don't have to read every detail on food labels to lose weight. Focus on total calories per serving to figure out what you're eating. (Calculate caloric density—number of calories per gram—by dividing the total calories per serving by the number of grams per serving.)

Just make sure you understand how the manufacturer defines a serving because sometimes it's half of what looks like a one-serving package. Watch out for deception that can wreck your efforts.

The Carb-Modified Diet encompasses all the best features of both low-carb and low-fat diets, and it also includes the new findings on when and what to eat for optimal weight management. With its five easy pieces and 4-3-2-1 pyramid, you'll find this plan easy to follow and flexible.

Now you won't have to get into diet controversies consuming Americans as women and men continue to eat and gain weight because they can't decipher what the experts say about what's the best macronutrient to put on their plates. Just for the record, the Carb-Modified Diet is low-fat (20 percent), high-protein (35–40 percent), and not low-carb (40–45 percent). The carb part is all about quality and timing.

The Fallacy of Phase 1

Fact #8: Deprivation is destructive to your diet.

It's reassuring to report that although there is much confusion and controversy about which diet works best, there's one area where all the experts agree: overly restrictive diets don't work. After an intense evaluation of dietary regimens, members of the National Institutes of Health's Nutrition Committee recommended caloric reduction in the moderate range, about 1,200 to 1,800 calories per day for most women and men who are 10 to 20 percent above their ideal body weight.

The committee denounced "very-low-calorie diets (VLCDs)," those that restrict you to four hundred to one thousand calories per day. Data on VLCDs show two major flaws:

- They are ineffective.
- They have very high dropout rates.

The Mogul Protocol discourages restrictive dieting practices from day one. This key feature sets it apart from many other diet programs. From my perspective, melba toast and cottage cheese, three-ounce protein servings, or eight-ounce meal replacements just don't work for long-term weight loss in most dieters older than age five.

With the addition of metformin, you get to skip the superstrict phase 1 that characterizes so many diets. And you avoid the very-low-calorie diet that the National Institutes of Health has panned. You don't need to give up fruits and carbohydrates to jump-start your metabolism or flush out fat to control those insulin spikes characteristic of Syndrome W (or any level of insulin resistance). Plus, you don't have to worry about gaining weight like you did when you "advanced" or moved past phase 1 of Atkins or South Beach Diet.

With the Mogul Protocol, concurrent use of medication targets and treats underlying insulin resistance and reduces hyperinsulinemia. So you don't need to suffer severe dietary deprivation to overcome the insulin elevations that trigger appetite when you eat forbidden fruits and starches. This expands your dietary options from day one of the diet and lets you focus on making those all-important long-term changes without severe food restriction in near starvation mode.

A second key feature of the Mogul Protocol is that "one" on the top of the 4-3-2-1 pyramid—the weekly treat. It's there to make sure you avoid the dietary deprivation and boredom that characterize the real-time weight loss of so many other diets. After the first month of the diet or the first five pounds lost, you get to enjoy a small piece of your cousin's birthday cake, your Aunt Polly's pecan pie, or your favorite restaurant's decadent fudge indulgence (but be sure you follow the rules on pages 88–89 to keep this "legal"). After you lose twenty-five pounds, or 10 to 15 percent of your initial body weight, and your insulin levels decline 30 to 50 percent, you will probably be able to expand your weekly treat to bi- or triweekly frequency.

The flexibility is one reason you'll find the Mogul Protocol easy to live with. And that's why so many of the women I've followed (some for more than a decade now) find the Carb-Modified Diet an easy and effective way to maintain long-term weight loss forever.

"Do" Dairy

Fact #9: Dairy foods can help you lose weight.

Just when we thought there was nothing new to say about food and diets, the data on dairy hit the headlines. As a longtime fan of dietary sources of micronutrients (vitamins and minerals), I tell my patients that little evidence suggests that taking a daily vitamin actually replicates the "benefits of the field."

We've spent millions of dollars analyzing diets and nutritional supplements in large populations of nurses, doctors, and samples of Americans, and the results show repeatedly that dietary supplements (antioxidants and other vitamins) fail to provide the health-enhancing effects of diets high in vegetables, fruits, fatty fishes, nuts, and such.

When the women I evaluate for obesity, osteoporosis, and other aging-related ailments ask, "What vitamins do you recommend?" my answer never varies; I always say "fruits and vegetables." Unless they have lactose intolerance (lack the enzyme that breaks down milk sugars), I encourage my patients to increase their calcium by consuming nonfat milk, low-fat dairy products, and other calcium-rich sources of dietary calcium (like green leafy vegetables, sardines, and fresh figs).

After a decade of promoting dietary calcium (specifically low-fat milk, yogurt, and cottage cheese) to my thin patients with osteoporosis and my overweight patients as a source of low-fat protein and other nutrients, I've been delighted to see the emerging research on dietary calcium and its recognition as the newest "anti-obesity" aid. As cited in a recent journal editorial, who could have imagined that calcium would attain such lofty status in just three years?

From old studies in children and adults, we knew that milk drinkers were less obese than their same-age peers, but experts attributed these findings to better overall diet, lack of snacking, and unmeasured traits of milk drinkers. But, in 2004, results were published from the first clinical trial of young adults randomized to calorie-restricted diets with placebo supplements, calcium-pill supplements, and increased dietary calcium sources. The group who got their calcium in their diets lost more weight and more inches from their waists than the group who took calcium supplements; both did better than the placebo-controlled group.

Liberal use of low-fat dairy products (two to three servings per day) in the Carb-Modified Diet differs from many other diet programs. Several popular diets devalue and delimit low-fat milk (sometimes in lieu of high-fat cream) because of milk "sugars." This recommendation is based on the invalid assumption that all simple sugars are metabolized equally and that they all trigger an undesirable release of insulin from the pancreas.

Now, state-of-the-art research from other centers supports the inclusion of low-fat dairy products. So I can continue to encourage dieters to add servings of no-sugar-added ice cream, low-carb ice-cream bars, and Equal- and Splenda-supplemented yogurt, all of which are widely available options and derivatives of the low-carb craze. These protein sources not only add variety to your diet but improve weight loss.

Diets Don't Work

Fact #10: Forget about diets to lose weight.

"Diet" is a word I try to avoid when helping women start a weight-loss program. Diets are on-again, off-again phenomena. Instead, I point to the "dietary component" of our program, and I focus on promoting long-term eating changes. Words are powerful agents for change, and the terms "flexible food plan" and "eating plan" more correctly reflect our philosophy. I don't believe in dieting.

A recent story in the "Styles" section of the *New York Times* featured celebrity waifs and doyennes of the under-forty fashion world who praised their favorite diets and diet gurus. Successful premenopausal dieters reported recent eating epiphanies, noting proudly that they were "on" Atkins or South Beach, Weight Watchers, or Jenny Craig. (Before that, it was Stillman or Scarsdale or the earliest version of Weight Watchers, the NYC Department of Health Diet.)

All of these diets reduce caloric intake and result in weight loss . . . in the short term, and there's the problem.

As any obesity expert will tell you, the big obstacle for weight-watching people is "long-term dietary adherence." What you need most is to be on "your own diet." You need to understand, once and for all, that there's absolutely nothing magical about a piece of paper, a brochure, or a book.

Let's be brutally honest here. When you contemplate going "on" the diet of the month, it signifies your not-so-unconscious intent of going "off" it at some yet-to-be-determined future point. Losing weight is a process—a series of learned skills. You need to develop a series of food choices and strategies for overcoming overeating in the real world of food. Hone those skills, and they're yours forever.

You'll find no simple substitute for the confidence you get from losing weight by creating your own dietary blueprint and using it to make changes in what and when you eat. Learning to eat correctly is just like learning to play a musical instrument, ride a bike, or ski a slope. You progress only with practice and coaching and the right tools. When you lose weight on the latest-greatest fad diet or by swilling powders or potions, you never acquire the necessary tools to keep those lost pounds off forever. *The Carb-Modified Diet is really not a "diet"—it's a lifestyle change!*

Summarizing and Synergizing

The Carb-Modified Diet provided on these pages is a healthy nutritional program that works for everyone but specifically targets women with insulin abnormalities.

This eating plan synergizes with metformin to reduce excess insulin levels, overcome Syndrome W, and ensure weight loss. Although developed long before the glycemic index (defined in 1981), the Carb-Modified Diet incorporates two of its important core concepts:

1. That increased food volume and fiber cut appetite and reverse weight gain
2. That large servings of vegetables and fruits are the easiest way to lose weight

This "nondiet" diet has worked for women in my practice for more than three decades, and it will work for you. Combine these large portions of vegetables and low-glycemic-index fruits with sizable portions of low-fat protein, two to three dairy products, and three starch servings each day, and you have plenty of food choices. You just need two key dietary changes to make this work:

- Change your breakfast menu.
- Cut out sandwiches for lunch.

Doable? Absolutely! That's why we call it the *five easy pieces*.

Now that you've learned nutrition 101 with all the latest updates, you're ready for more details of the diet component of the Mogul Protocol.

Chapter 20

ADDING BEHAVIOR MODIFICATION
TO CARBOHYDRATE MODIFICATION

Replacing Old Habits
with New and Better Ones

MAKING LIFESTYLE CHANGES INVOLVES a bit of behavior modification in some of our patients. If you are classic and early Syndrome W— only twenty pounds to go to get back into your size 10s—you can skip this chapter. If you've been almost effortlessly thin or normal-weight all your life and never overate until you were derailed by the consequences of hyperinsulinemia after Syndrome W struck, all you need are the Mogul Protocol's Carb-Modified Diet and metformin. You will almost certainly succeed in shedding those newly accumulated pounds. You'll probably easily become another testimony to the benefits of early identification and treatment of Syndrome W.

But if you've been somewhat overweight or obese lifelong and have experienced additional weight surges in your forties or fifties, your story is slightly different. Baseline weight—your weight when you're first diagnosed with Syndrome W—turns out to be an important predictor of how well the diet and medication will work. We discovered this when we looked at women in two different weight groups (overweight and obese) in our metformin study. One reason for this difference was the higher percentage of problem eating behaviors reported by higher-weight women.

Our patients in higher-weight categories did very well. In fact, as a group, they lost more weight, with a more dramatic change from their beginning weight. But they needed a few more treatment visits in the first year (seven to eight compared with five for the other women) and a slightly higher dose of medication to reduce hunger and food cravings. They all had to change the following behaviors:

- Fast eating
- Stress-related eating
- Lapses from diet

Working with these women, we developed effective tools and techniques that help to make this book a manual for change.

If you weigh more than 200 pounds, have a body mass index greater than 32, and/or have a history of binge eating, however YOU define it, this chapter is critical reading.

The Behavior Modification Revolution: Then and Now

Albert Stunkard's early-1980s research in the eating disorders program at the University of Pennsylvania challenged traditional dietary treatments for obesity. These pioneering studies showed that behavior modification worked better than caloric restriction in helping people lose weight and keep it off. Clinical trials showed that research subjects who restructured their eating behaviors lost more weight and regained fewer pounds than did their counterparts who received diet alone. Follow-up data two years later showed that more than 90 percent of patients who were treated with a program of behavior modification maintained their weight loss, whereas 95 percent of patients who received only a weight-reducing diet during the treatment phase regained all the weight they had lost and more.

Dr. Stunkard's behavior-modification techniques were published in a textbook for health-care professionals called the LEARN Program, later adapted for workbooks by the American Diabetes Association. With the exception of the excellent book *Thin Tastes Better*, by New York City psychologist Robert Gullo, PhD, a simple guide to the basics of behavior modification, there were few ideas on behavior mod 101 available to the dieting public for many years. A new book, *The Beck Diet Solution*, by psychologist Judith Beck, provides additional detail for restructuring eating behaviors.

Today, primary care physicians receive no training in helping patients modify behaviors, but you can do it yourself (DIY) with a few good sources. Learn about the LEARN Program so that you can adopt these useful strategies for permanent weight loss. You may even want to share them with your physician. The following are some behavior-modification ideas that you can start using immediately.

Journal Your Eating

Your eating patterns are revealing. They speak to your priorities, personality, attitudes, and values. And the more familiar you become with your modus operandi at the dinner table, restaurants, parties, celebrations—even in the car, the subway, or walking down the street, wherever and whenever you eat—the easier time you'll have putting the Mogul Protocol to work for you.

You can benefit greatly from keeping eating records. Collate them into a food diary as a way to scrutinize your eating activities. A food journal can serve as a foolproof way to tally food, fullness ratings, and other aspects of your eating. When beginning the Mogul Protocol, food records are especially helpful because they accelerate weight loss as your eating becomes a conscious act and you raise your awareness of mindless eating.

After only a few days of journaling, you'll see patterns emerge. You can learn the following:

- What and who trigger you to overeat
- Where and when things go off course

This knowledge will help you get past obstacles. Eating records are an invaluable aid for altering lifelong habits that cause us to overeat. Be sure to add them to your arsenal.

The food diary (page 139), developed to monitor research subjects, calls for an estimate of portion size when you're charting intake. Each triangle represents one serving so that you can keep track of your progress and your tally every day. You also give yourself a check if you eat "correctly" based on the guidelines for healthy eating behaviors. You even record your eight glasses of water a day and log your daily exercise and activities.

Check It Out

Here's my list of "Standard Stunkard," which is my version of the guidelines for weight loss first published during the behavior modification revolution. These are simple but important guidelines that can help you change destructive eating behaviors and promote long-term weight loss.

Notice the columns in the food diary. These allow you to keep tabs on those eating behaviors that can compromise the best intentions. Put a check mark in the box if you've been successful. See "My Food Diary" and the "Sample Food Diary" and the descriptions below to guide you.

Eat Sitting Down—Not Standing Up

Make a check mark in column 1 in the food diary if you did this. You can eliminate overeating if you vow that you'll never, ever eat while:

- Standing up
- Peering into your refrigerator
- Walking out the door
- Sitting/lying in bed at night
- Preparing meals
- Cleaning up after meals

All these "positions" lead to mindless eating. Believe it or not, you can consume thousands of calories if you snack while answering your e-mail, baking cookies, or sampling hors d'oeuvres. You won't even notice because mindless eating isn't a conscious act.

Focus on Your Food When You Eat

Don't mix eating with another activity. (See "Focus," column 2 of the food diary.) In an era defined by multitasking, it's very tempting to try to save time by eating while you do something else—watch your kids, read the newspaper, surf the Net. This may add a little extra time to your schedule, but it will also add many extra calories each day and extra pounds each year. This isn't ideal for either time management *or* weight management. It's another route to mindless eating.

Slow Down and Taste the Food

(See "Slow" and "Taste," columns 3 and 4 in the food diary.) You would be surprised how many minutes it takes for fullness signals from the

My Food Diary

Name: S M T W Th F S   **Date:**

TIME	FOOD / BEVERAGE	SIT DOWN	FOCUS	SLOW	TASTE	HUNGER FULLNESS RATING 1-10	MOOD FEELINGS (DESCRIBE)
	Breakfast						
	Lunch						
	4 p.m. Snack						
	Dinner						
	Other snack (optional)						
	Weekly treat (after 1 month or as indicated)						

Total number of pills today: none Δ   1 Δ   2 Δ   3 Δ   4 Δ

Food Plan:

		Exercise:	
Proteins	Δ Δ Δ Δ	Walk	Δ
Vegetables (min)	Δ Δ Δ Δ	Run	Δ
Fruits	Δ Δ Δ	Dance and movement	Δ
Starches	Δ Δ Δ	Fitness class	Δ
Fats	Δ Δ	Other_____	Δ
Dairy Servings	Δ Δ		
Water/Non-caloric beverages	Δ Δ Δ Δ Δ Δ Δ Δ	Total Time_____ minutes	

My Food Diary

My Food Diary

Name:		S M T W Th F S				Date: 7/19/05	

TIME	FOOD / BEVERAGE	SIT DOWN	FOCUS	SLOW	TASTE	HUNGER FULLNESS	MOOD FEELINGS (DESCRIBE)
	Breakfast	√			√	6	Rushed
7 a.m.	3 egg-white omelet with mushrooms, peppers						Read paper
	1 cup berries						
	coffee with 1% milk						
	Lunch	√	√	√	√	8	Enjoyed meal
12:30	Large salad with 1 cup mixed chopped veggies						Felt satisfied
	4-oz. skinless chicken breast						
	Dressing: 1-oz. olive oil w/ 2T balsamic vinegar						
	18-oz. coffee – milkshake (skim milk /n Splenda)						
	4 p.m. Snack	√		√	√	8	
4:15	1 Diet Snapple						
	1 1-oz. package lite (e.g. Boston Light) popcorn						
	1 string cheese						
	Dinner	√	√	√	√	8	No deprivation
7 p.m.	6-oz. grilled salmon with mustard sauce						Couldn't finish
	1 cup broccoli						
	grilled red peppers, onions, zucchini						
	½ cup brown rice pilaf						
	large salad with low-calorie dressing						
	6-oz. glass dry white wine						
	1 serving frozen low-fat yogurt with 1 cup berries						
	Other snack (optional)						
	1 orange						
	Weekly treat (after 1 month or as indicated)	√	√	√	√	8	Really enjoyed
10 p.m.	1 small slice birthday cake						GREAT!!!

Total number of pills today: none Δ   1 Δ   2 Δ   3 Δ   4 Δ

Food Plan:		Exercise	
Proteins	Δ Δ Δ	Walk	Δ
Vegetables (min)	Δ Δ ΔΔ	Run	Δ
Fruits	Δ Δ Δ	Dance and movement	Δ
Starches	Δ Δ Δ	Fitness class	Δ
Fats	Δ Δ	other_____	Δ
Dairy Servings	Δ Δ		
Water/Non-caloric beverages	Δ Δ Δ Δ Δ Δ Δ Δ	total time_____ minutes	

My Food Diary

gut and GI tract to tell you it's time to stop eating. That's just one more good reason you should try not to rush through meals. Seek to recapture the dinner of yesteryear, which is fast becoming a dinosaur—times when families dined together and talked and used this as a bonding experience. Departures from the sit-down dinner have led to the fast-food and fast-feeding frenzy that make you and your family eat more than you used to.

If your hand is in perpetual motion between "cup and lip," try these helpful strategies:

- Don't let your eating be one nonstop motion. Put your fork down between bites until you have finished each forkful. Don't gulp food. Use that time to chew slowly and become more aware of what you're eating before you swallow. Sadly, fast-food burgers and tenders are so pulverized that you don't even have to chew before you swallow.
- Mix up your eating utensils. Use chopsticks. They'll make you eat smaller bites at a slower pace. If you eat with one hand in the American tradition, follow the cues of our less-obese European friends and use both hands: fork in left hand (if you're right-handed), knife in the right hand. Before going public, practice this first at home with a napkin on your lap. After you've mastered the technique, you'll see how much slower you eat and how much more you enjoy food.
- Give up finger food. Use a fork for everything you're used to eating by hand. Cutting tidbits you would usually pop in your mouth is a good way to stretch calories and make eating more mindful. This may make eating at parties tougher, and if so, that's great! Most social gatherings have a place to sit down, plate in hand, so that you can savor those savories. Change the way you eat chicken tenders, chunks of cheese, crudités with dip, tacos and nachos, and especially the (allowable) sandwiches and slices of pizza. Keep your fingers clean while you cut back on calories.
- Use your left hand (if you're right-handed) for everything else. Grapes, almonds, popcorn, and pretzels last longer if you eat them one morsel at a time with your nondominant (other than usually used) hand.
- Cut your food into small pieces. Instructions on the Heimlich maneuver are displayed in restaurants because people really do choke on the big portions they put in their mouths. (In some

states, health courses that teach the Heimlich maneuver are a requirement for high school graduation. This is because health officials recognize the health hazards of large bites. They are bad for short-term as well as long-term health.)

Figure Out Whether You're Full and How You Feel

Last are those all-important final two columns in the food diary. Here's where you tally the mind-meal connection that we now know underlies why we start and stop eating. The simplest way to do this is to use a ten-point scale where 1 = starving, that truly famished "can't wait to get home and get to the refrigerator" state when you haven't had a minute to eat all day, and 10 = groaningly, painfully, post-Thanksgiving-feast full. Your goal here is to stay midzone and avoid the pain of both extremes. Finally, use a few shortcut terms and jot down how you feel after you've finished eating. Food records may seem simplistic, but some of my savviest patients are surprised at the insights they can supply on the road to lifetime weight-loss maintenance.

Graze Not, Grab Not

Limit your consumption of trigger foods. Cookies, chips, candy, and even "healthy" bites based on protein, air, and additives all lead to overeating because you can't eat just one. These are high in calories, and most are high in trans fats, which damage coronary arteries and increase your risk of heart disease. Nuts, cheese, trail mix, and granola look more benign, but they also spell trouble. Get these out of your cupboards and off your list permanently.

Join a Group

You may find it useful to attend a diet and nutrition workshop or behavior modification group sponsored by local community or commercial weight-reduction organizations. They offer a useful forum for discussion of weight issues. The workshops crystallize key problems. When one voice at a conference room table describes an experience or stumbling block and you see many heads nodding synchronously in agreement, you know you've hit a common chord for collective resolution. Certain subjects come up over and over again. They are the themes that dominate the weight struggles of all women, of all ages and all ethnicities.

What stressors cause weight gain? What life events trigger upward weight and downward mood spirals? Which behaviors help and which hinder weight loss?

What's the most prevalent theme of all? The one that always heads the list at such discussions? Here's the key, the sine qua non for success, learned from all those patient dialogues: the important decision of making "me time."

Make Yourself a Priority

The single most important thing you will need to do is figure out how to get on your to-do list. The book *Fat Is a Feminist Issue* (reissued 1997), by Susie Orbach, made this a crusade twenty years ago. And, according to current surveys, women two decades ago actually had more time than women today do, and that goes for all activities: child rearing, meal preparation, socializing, leisure time, and even sleep time.

An increasing number of American women work both outside and inside the home. And despite technological advances meant to make life flow more efficiently, at the end of the (long) day, most women list time as the one thing they lack that's needed to make the lifestyle changes required for that New Year's resolution to get and stay fit.

All the women we see are overcommitted and underappreciated. They all put themselves way down on their "tasks" list. The nurses who make up 10 percent of my practice are typical women in that respect. They spend all day nurturing others but rarely take time to nurture themselves. This is easily the number one flaw of women who fail to lose weight when they try otherwise effective remedies.

If your insulin curve shows that you have hyperinsulinemia, your need for medication and weight loss is more than theoretical. Hyperinsulinemia is early evidence that you're on a path to serious and significant disease. This is your wake-up call. Use this information as an impetus to make treatment a top priority. Understand that the Mogul Protocol can halt the progression of Syndrome W into Syndrome X and diabetes and that you are past the point for postponements. Forget those maybes. Put yourself on the list, and make it "me time" this time. You will need to set aside thirty minutes a day to promote weight loss and prevent diabetes and heart disease. That's the bare minimum, but it is nonnegotiable.

Use this time for fifteen minutes of exercise and fifteen minutes of meal planning/preparation each day. The first week of your Mogul

Protocol efforts, you will also need to block out several hours to clean out your pantry and restock your shelves and your refrigerator with new staples: fresh (or frozen) vegetables, fruits, low-fat dairy products, soups, and fresh or frozen food products to supply protein and variety for modular meal planning (see chapter 18).

If you can't find the thirty minutes daily, you have two choices:

- Do less each day.
- Delegate chores at home or work.
- Decrease the number of hours you sleep each night. (This may not be a good option since recent research shows that sleep deprivation, fewer than six hours of sleep per night, is associated with weight gain!)

Bottom line, it's up to you to make it work.

Chapter 21

STAYING ON TRACK EVERYWHERE YOU GO

Ways to Guard against Slip-Sliding Away

BE PREPARED AND ANTICIPATE OBSTACLES to healthy eating so you're not caught off guard. Here are a few simple guidelines to avoid slipups that could evolve into big transgressions.

Use the Low-Fat Latte Secret
When You're Short of Time

One not-so-secret ingredient of my diet is my staple—the low-fat (skim-milk) latte. I discovered its power while giving my first major scientific presentation at the International Endocrine Society meeting in 1996.

Eighteen thousand attended the meeting at the Moscone Convention Center in San Francisco, where the attendees heard five days of experts' presentations. Sessions started at 6:30 a.m. and ran into the night. I had to make tough choices because there was so much to see and do. So I got up early each morning and stopped at Starbucks for a low-fat latte on the way to and from the meetings. Faced with long lines at lunch-food concessions and long waits for tables at nearby restaurants, I simply had another latte at lunch and then kept going, cramming in as many sessions as possible. I learned more than endocrinology from this experience.

To my great astonishment, I found that when I got back to my hotel room, I wasn't a bit hungry, despite fourteen hours without solid foods! Even when I joined colleagues for dinner at SF's finest food emporia, I wasn't inclined to overeat. What amazed me was how this differed from prior occasions. Usually, when I'd skipped lunch to deal with medical or other emergencies at the office, I was totally famished by late afternoon, and I experienced true physical hunger.

At first, I just dismissed my "latte diet" in San Francisco as an aberration; after all, it was an amazing panorama of science and my first scientific presentation, so I assumed I was just a bit revved up on adrenaline. Then I began to think about some old and very important data on protein.

In the early 1970s, George Blackburn, director of nutrition at Harvard, advocated the liquid-protein-sparing fast as a strategy to avoid excess muscle breakdown in patients who were undergoing starvation treatment for life-threatening obesity. The initial preparation was a solution of amino acids (proteins) with added flavoring. Liquid protein supplements later became available for use as meal substitutes under a variety of brand names, and they're still used today in some weight-loss programs at leading medical institutions. Presenters at a 2004 meeting of the North American Obesity Society demonstrated that products such as Optifast can play a role in promoting long-term weight control in certain people.

I mulled it over and realized that skim milk was, of course, just a solution of amino acids. So a low-fat latte was simply a very tasty form of liquid protein with a bit of caffeine added, which, presumably, had reversed my loss of energy from food deprivation during the late afternoon.

I generally advocate other sources of protein, plus vegetables and some fruit as the ideal breakfast and lunch combo. But if you don't have time to sit down and eat proper meals at these times, lattes are a great way to prevent starvation and keep going all day.

Milk, as we know, is one of nature's perfect foods, with its high content of vitamins and minerals. Large studies show that American children who are milk drinkers are less likely to be obese than their non-milk-drinking classmates. Similarly, Scandinavian adults with higher dietary calcium intake weigh less than countrymates who consume less calcium in their diets. The most recent data have shown that adding calcium via dairy products to a low-cal diet helps with weight loss.

It may surprise you to learn that two sixteen-ounce lattes (twenty-four ounces of milk) a day can supply almost two-thirds of the daily calcium requirement for women, and it comes in a form that may be better for bone health than calcium from tablets.

One more bonus from the four ounces of coffee in that grande-sized latte is coffee's protective effect in preventing diabetes. Hot off the press in December 2009 are the results of a large study detailing the relationship between the number of cups of coffee (decaf or regular) consumed each day with a reduction in the risk of diabetes. Bravo espresso!

These days, I always keep a low-fat latte on my desk. It's my signature drink. I order it extra hot and then take sips in between patients, while making notes during my office hours. You can get low-fat lattes caffeinated or decaffeinated, with nonsugar vanilla syrup or with soy milk (if you're lactose intolerant).

If you have no time for Starbucks, make the following brew to go. Here's the scoop:

Start with 12–16 ounces skim milk or soy milk—warm in the microwave.

Add 1–2 tablespoons instant coffee or double tea bag or (if you like neither) 1–2 ounces non-sugar-added vanilla, raspberry, dulce de leche, or hazelnut syrup (widely available).

Now there are no more excuses for skipping breakfast!

Finesse Your Restaurant Forays

Because we eat more than one-third of our meals outside of our homes, restaurant survival tactics come in handy. The fact is, restaurant eating can actually add an extra measure of control and make it easier to lose weight. When you eat most of your meals at home, you can inadvertently underestimate the dimension of your dinner; so there can be better portion control eating out (if you're careful in your calculation).

Also, turning over the kitchen to someone else can decrease stress and encourage you to linger and chat (rarely the case with home-front meals). This makes the occasion more conversation oriented than food oriented, which is a good thing for your eating plan.

Here are some helpful dining-out tips:

- Don't go anywhere hungry. Always take along a piece of fruit or a 100-calorie snack and lots of fluid.
- Drink plenty of tap or bottled water while you're waiting for your food to arrive.
- Limit yourself to one small roll or slice of bread, and then ask the waiter to remove the bread basket.

- Choose the right restaurants. Go to diet-friendly eateries. Although you can make good selections in most cuisines, some categories give you more leeway than others. For the Carb-Modified Diet, you'll find the most options at seafood and American food restaurants. You can have grilled fish, broiled seafood, and chicken breasts, to name just a few low-calorie options. Italian and Japanese eateries (especially those with sushi bars) are your second line of priority. Chinese, Indian, and Mexican are trickier because it's hard to estimate the oil content when an entrée has multiple ingredients.
- Don't open the menu. Figure out what you're going to eat before you get there, and ask for exactly that. No problem! Make reasonable requests and reasonable substitutions. Remember Meg Ryan in *When Harry Met Sally*? She singlehandedly made it cool to special-order. You can easily just ask the waiter to give you sauce or dressing on the side, a double serving of vegetables in place of the starch, and "light on the oil" for mixed-ingredient main courses and sides. The majority of restaurants today offer healthy alternatives because they work to try to keep customers happy. Many restaurateurs have added "light" options in all categories.
- Stick with what works—the foolproof "formula" for dinner:

    Appetizer: Have seafood, noncream soup, green salad, or a vegetable. (Choose one of the side veggies if none is under appetizers.)

    Entrée: Choose fish, chicken, or just about any other grilled or roasted item.

    Starch: Avoid unless it's steamed rice or grains.

    Vegetables: Ask for extras and order them steamed or "light on the oil or butter."

    Dessert: Order one for the table and have a spoonful, or use as your "weekly treat."

- Take home a doggie bag to limit your excess and help with portion control. This is now acceptable at the chicest restaurants.

Ban Buffets (or Manhandle Them)

Few absolutes exist in a lifelong strategy for weight control, but one exception is the buffet. Don't go there! Buffets can derail the most focused dieters. But if you understand your motivations, you can be better equipped to deter dysfunctional eating at buffets.

Here are some of the "issues" for unwary eaters facing buffet tables:

- *We feel a strong urge to indulge because the meal is all-inclusive.* Our capitalist values and bargain-seeking "inner selves" reinforce the notion that the more we eat, the more we are getting for our money.
- *Seeing large portions makes it hard to apply portion control.* Most buffets provide an unparalleled opportunity to heap our plates.
- *We're taken in by captivating presentations.* In addition to sheer quantity and variety, the food is presented so beautifully that it's especially tempting.
- *We have no server/gatekeeper to hold us back; it's a dining free-for-all.* Without Big Brother, it's easy to overload your plate.
- *The theme of a buffet centers on what you avoid, not what you consume.* You can easily excuse your gluttony by saying, "Oh, but I didn't eat the chocolate mousse or the bananas Foster!"
- *You enjoy the festivities and the camaraderie of other diners, and eating just seems so right.* Peer pressure definitely promotes excessive eating because we hear other people touting their discoveries ("You must try the coconut shrimp—they're fabulous!") and excuse their overindulgence ("I'll make up for this lasagna at the gym on Monday!").

Moving Right Along

Of course, you can move right on past the buffet tables—that's one excellent solution. And you can opt for a meal that works better for you; many hotels have à la carte options for those who don't like buffets. Also, you can ask for the chef to make you an egg-white omelet, a salad, or grilled fish.

If You Just Have to Queue Up

If you do decide to visit the buffet, here are some tips for negotiating the experience without abandoning your Carb-Modified Diet:

- *Check out what's offered before you pick up your plate.* Many buffets have salads, vegetables, and low-fat protein dishes. So if you first pile your plate with mayonnaise-laden, high-fat appetizers and richly sauced pastas, you won't have room for the grilled vegetables or salmon fillets at the end of the table.

- *Find a surrogate server to fetch your food so that you don't have to cruise the full array of options.* Give your buffet buddy a short list; you want
    - Fish or seafood appetizer
    - Lots of green salad and one spoonful (not ladleful) of the lowest-cal dressing
    - Vegetables
    - One or two choices of low-fat protein
    - One tablespoon of a single high-calorie item (penne in vodka, hash-brown potatoes, turkey stuffing)—to perk up your plate
- *Make it a personal rule that you will never go back for seconds.*
- *Plan a single "spoonful of sugar" or a plateful of fruit for that sweet-tooth finale.* Ask a friend or a waiter to retrieve it. Order your end-of-meal beverage first (coffee, tea, espresso, cappuccino), and after it comes, pick that one "poison" (unless you opted for the fruit plate).

Follow these buffet strategies, and you'll do fine. Plus, you won't walk away feeling lethargic and stuffed like everyone else.

Car Safety

Texting while driving is now verboten, but eating en route is increasingly accepted. Some rules of the road will help.

Food is a distraction, and consuming a complete meal while behind the wheel is frankly dangerous. However, it won't hurt to have a snack on your long commute homeward. Just keep it small and simple. Eat an apple and drink a diet soda or sip a low-calorie tea to cut your appetite in the late afternoon. Keep an orange in the car (peel it before you hit the traffic) and cans of V8 in the trunk, and store a one-ounce package of pretzels, string cheese, or cheddar cheese.

This minimeal on your way home can help you avoid excess snacking and tasting rampages while you're preparing dinner. Plus, the boost you get from that extra 150 calories will make you less grumpy and more likable when you arrive home and greet your family. (Starvation mode is rarely a win-friends-influence-people modus operandi.)

Prevent Party Pitfalls

You also must be prepared for the most taste-tempting part of the year—the holidays, when many Americans pack on ten to fifteen pounds with the best of excuses—we can't hurt people's feelings when they're offering us Thanksgiving/Christmas food!

In fact, this is such a problem for people who are watching their weight that our clinic gives out party survival handouts that reflect certain times of the year: bright orange at Thanksgiving, bright red and green at Christmas, and lavender at Easter. We use colors to explain the diet game to some of our very young patients and those who have developmental disabilities. The following is our one-page summary of strategies that help people manage to celebrate holiday festivities without going too far off course. Having these in hand will help you celebrate during and after the holidays.

Tips for Partygoers

- *Use bright hues as your guide to correct food choices. Think red, green, and orange*—even blue and purple. Most vegetables and fruits in these colors are low in calories and healthy. An added bonus: most are high in antioxidants, which protect against heart disease, cancer, and the ravages of aging. Red, green, blue, orange, and purple are keys to healthy eating for all meals and especially handy if you keep these hues in mind when you attend holiday gatherings.
- *Think bad brown and worse white.* Other than mushrooms, most *brown* items at parties are a problem. All those puffs, potato pancakes, fritters, pigs-in-a-blanket, crab cakes, Chinese egg rolls, little pizzas, deep-fried vegetables (tempura), fried clams, and meatballs are filled with calories, about one hundred a bite. *Avoid all nuts* (several hundred calories per handful). *Watch out for white foods/beverages:* mayo-laden dips, brie, eggnog, ice cream, cream cheese, whipped cream, snowballs, bacon-wrapped tidbits. (But turkey and fish are fine.)
- *Remember that cheese is essentially fat, so show restraint* when eating baked brie and cheese cubes. About one ounce of cheese, which is the size of a domino, equals 90 to 120 calories.
- *Don't go out hungry. Have a piece of fruit or a hundred-calorie healthy snack (a cup of air-popped popcorn is perfect).*

- *Walk around with a "drink" in your hand.* You can have Perrier, club soda, Diet Coke, Pepsi, or Fresca, with ice, lemon, or lime; a "Virgin Mary" (Bloody Mary mix, V8 juice, or tomato juice); or Diet 7-Up or club soda with a splash of grapefruit, orange, or cranberry juice.
- *Avoid standing near food.* It's so easy just to position yourself far away from platters, punch bowls, and buffet table. Don't go near the kitchen or spots where waiters are passing hot canapés.
- *Survey the scene and time your eating.* Find low-cal items to munch on. Good choices are crudités (watch the dip), shrimp and other seafood, sushi, vegetable rolls (California rolls), and small amounts of grilled beef or chicken (e.g., teriyaki). Stuffed mushrooms are good. Naturally, you want to select fresh fruit over cookies. Plan to have one special cookie or a small taste (a tablespoon) of dessert just before leaving.
- *Practice saying "no thank you."* Visualize yourself saying this.
- *Enjoy good company!* Focus on the people who are there; that makes you a better party person, and you won't eat out of boredom or just because the food exists.
- *Dance if there's music.* This is a great way to burn up calories and have fun!

Be a Forearmed Road Warrior

Increased airport security, airline delays, anxious fellow passengers, and understaffed airlines now create extra stress that takes its toll on your diet resolve. Plan ahead to avoid trouble, whether you're flying, sailing, or going Amtrak.

Your best approach is identifying all dietary demons:

- *Temper the terminal food.* Food courts and food concessions are not safe havens. Spend a few extra minutes to look for healthy alternatives to cookie shops and pizza parlors. Seek out seafood bars and grills that offer chicken breasts and salads. If you have a hamburger or pizza, top it smartly: mushrooms, onions, lettuce/tomato, but no bacon or cheese as an add-on. If the only sides are fries, onion rings, chips, and beans, substitute salad or salsa. Unwrap the wrap you bought; remove the tortilla. Or order it "bare" if they're not premade.

- *Steer clear of extra food choices.* Cut back temporarily on your allowable three daily starches because you won't have the regular options available when you travel. "None" may be easier than "some." You may find it simpler on trips to change modes; opt for a diet of protein, fruit, and vegetables only. Travel offers strong temptations at breakfast buffets, coffee shops, and dessert tables. Have your mind made up to just say no. But do treat yourself to your favorite dessert on the trip home to celebrate how well you did with your new self-control.

- *Say thanks but no thanks to alcohol.* Although the three-martini lunch is a relic of the past, alcohol is still omnipresent at business dinners, conferences, conventions, and cruises. Whether you're looking at little bottles on planes or in your hotel room minibar, you know that alcohol flows freely on trips, so you need a game plan to cling to.

  If you meet someone for a drink, ask for Diet Coke. Remember, many of today's chic mixed drinks are full of calories. So they do double damage by hurting your dietary vigilance and adding to your day's calories. Good alternatives to diet soda when you have to have a drink in your hand? Try a Virgin Mary, white wine spritzer with extra club soda and ice, or light beer.

- *Tweak business dinners your own way.* To avoid being at the mercy of meal planners, take some control of what's under those shiny domes. Find a waiter, and ask for a few modifications: a salad in place of an appetizer, a double order of vegetables, or maybe a fish entrée. You won't be an oddity; diners are getting more assertive all the time at pre-fixed dinners. Don't apologize for eating healthy. Just stick with what's good for you. You matter!

- *Take exercise breaks.* Pack sneakers and workout shorts so that you'll make a break in your schedule for staying fit. Most hotel chains have gyms on-site. You can go online beforehand and find out what amenities your hotel has. Then pack accordingly. If you can't do your usual exercise, download an exercise tape or take to the streets around your hotel. Make exercise a part of your business day.

- *Fight fatigue with power naps.* A nap of about thirty minutes can help combat travel fatigue from extra work hours, decreased sleep, and jet lag. Tune into the airline's earphones, take along a headset for your handheld, or pack your iPod so that you can listen to relaxing music. Slow your breathing, clear your mind, and reduce stress en route and back. It's a good idea to find a way to handle travel fatigue, which often leads to mindless eating.

Chapter 22

ALL THINGS AEROBIC AND A BIT OF HERESY

Exercise If You Can

EVENTUALLY, AFTER DISCUSSING metabolism, medication, and diet, my patients always ask, "What about exercise?"

I think about exercise a lot. Having been a "jock" at a time when women in sports were an anomaly, I'm fortunate to have had a lifelong interest in exercise, which, by the way, has not always translated to exercise participation. In my early career as director of student health services at Barnard College, I worked closely with the Department of Physical Education and Dance to promote healthy exercise in young women. As the official team physician first for Barnard and later for Columbia women, I spent countless hours at meetings with coaches, trainers, and sports-medicine orthopedists trying to figure out what works best for women. The truth is, we know only a little more now than we knew then. But *I've always been a firm believer in exercise for overall health.* I'm convinced it serves many purposes, including the following evidence-based effects:

- Reverses the ravages of aging
- Lowers of the risk of diabetes and heart disease
- Enhances mind and body functions
- Reduces blood pressure
- Improves your level of good cholesterol
- Decreases depression
- Imparts a sense of empowerment
- Wards off hot flashes

Some studies show that regular exercise may decrease your likelihood of developing breast cancer if you start working out when you're young.

Getting Real

However, I must admit that I'm also a bit of a heretic when it comes to endorsing exercise as an answer for weight management in women. I know this view is counter to conventional wisdom, but I promise it's based on conversations with my patients and the somewhat surprising conclusions from several large clinical trials of exercise in women. **That's why I don't insist on having an exercise "prong" to the Mogul Protocol. I'm just not comfortable giving advice that could keep women from trying the other two critical components of the plan because they think they have to commit to aerobic conditioning and can't see themselves following through with an exercise regimen.**

What Women Want and Need to Know

Here are the problems I've observed over the years:

Women don't like to exercise, and they hate to sweat.

I've talked with hundreds of women about exercise—inner-city women participating in our menopause program in New York City; CEO commuters from Chappaqua, New York; adolescents and octogenarians; women from affluent suburbs and ghettos and all strata of society and life circumstance. Their message is loud and clear. "We hate to exercise," they all say, and they really mean it. Even my precollege elite athletes, in the privacy of the exam room, complain about the boredom of basketball training and confide that they would sometimes rather be at the mall than on the field. Women are sidetracked for many reasons. Some say that it's the safety of the neighborhood or the inability to afford a desirable program; others simply face the fact that they really don't enjoy walking on a treadmill, step machine, or elliptical trainer. I see so many women who have bicycles in their basements, hand weights in their attics, and unused gym memberships. And I've watched hundreds of overweight women struggle to become more active with little success. This contrasts dramatically with my overweight male patients, who usually integrate exercise into their lives rather effortlessly, making regular workouts part of their weight-loss programs.

Biology Is Destiny

Aerobic exercise doesn't help women lose weight.

Many women have tried aerobic exercise to shed pounds and have grown frustrated when it didn't work. This stems from the unfortunate gender difference that exists regarding the effect of exercise on weight loss in women compared with men. While exercise is clearly a key factor in helping men shed pounds, producing significant and sustainable body weight loss even without drastic dietary change, most studies of women show that exercise alone doesn't produce meaningful weight loss.

Studies in which women are "randomized" (assigned to treatment with an exercise regimen or diet program or both) reveal that women who do regular, intense, monitored exercise alone don't lose a significant amount of weight after six months (in contrast to women who follow the prescribed dietary program); also, women who both diet and exercise lose no more weight than women who diet exclusively. Studies of young college athletes and older wannabe athletes also show that vigorous exercise regimens do not lead to significant weight loss in females unless they work out many times (five or more) a week *or* they also diet. Most of these studies defined exercise in the aerobic mode. A few new studies demonstrate that weight training can help glucose control in diabetics and may also help weight loss in combination with diet or a program of aerobic conditioning.

Exercise Can Help Women Maintain Their Weight

On the other hand, several studies suggest that regular exercise may benefit *weight maintenance* for women. There is growing evidence that women who exercise (after losing weight) have less weight "regain" than women who don't.

Finally, a recent study indicates that the amount of weight women gain each year is directly related to how little (or how much) they exercise and the intensity of their workouts. It appears that regular exercise allows women to eat a little bit more each day without reaccumulating pounds. Working out also lets you broaden your food choices and serves as an excellent indicator of long-term success. You'll see the careful eater/exerciser prevail every time. Then, of course, there are those all-important, less-tangible benefits of exercise—stress reduction and mood elevation, which can go a long way to help limit excess eating and stabilize weight.

What We Don't Know about the Weight/Exercise Link

No studies explain the exercise gender gap; why workouts help men lose weight but are less effective for women has not been adequately addressed with research. We can speculate that it may be due to men's higher levels of testosterone, which help to build muscle and thereby improve "resting energy expenditure"—calories burned at rest. Or it may be due to innate body composition or other hormonal differences. We can't expect to modify these factors—level the playing field—until we have a better understanding of why women are not more like men on and off the courts.

Getting Rhythm and Motion

So here's the bottom line. *Make exercise a part of your day—if you can! Be honest about what you're doing and what you're likely to do.* That's the best way to integrate exercise into the Mogul Protocol as part of a long-term lifestyle change for a healthier, slimmer life.

Some Tips for an Individualized Approach

- *Exercise if you can. Don't feel guilty if you can't.* Don't worry or get down on yourself if you're not ready to start exercising. If you're already overcommitted and results oriented, don't add guilt over your lack of exercise. Instead, *start with changing your diet and modifying your eating behaviors, and as you lose weight, you'll find yourself becoming receptive to the idea of getting into a bathing suit to swim or tights to spin.* Think about simple ways to increase your activity level, but don't feel "pushed" to participate in formal exercise programs until you're all systems go. The Mogul Protocol is very much antiguilt.
- *Set realistic expectations.* Women are sometimes more unrealistic about the effects of exercise than men. We cheer for the week's greatest losers on those reality TV shows, and we're overly susceptible to the media blitz in late December. You know those shots of bikini-clad nymphets frolicking in the sand, followed by a split-screen image of women working out en masse in a

health club. The message is that gym membership in January guarantees perfect biceps and buns of steel by July; you just get in there and do forty-five minutes, three times a week, and you'll look like Britney.

These pie-in-the-sky promises don't help, of course, because you end up demoralized when your mirror image in July is only slightly better than the one in January. The fact is, even actress Hilary Swank, preparing to play a boxer in *Million Dollar Baby*, had to put in three to four gym hours a day to hone her impressive musculature. Even the newest health guidelines do a great disservice to women, calling for ninety minutes a day of exercise. I suspect you can't spare that kind of time each day, and it's really okay.

- *Do the math—right.* Don't overestimate your calories burned. Some women have a tough time calculating the number of calories burned in a forty-five-minute walk or a ninety-minute tennis match. And that's despite the fact that we see exercise charts with calories burned per hour per activity on the walls of most health clubs. The truth is, many activities just don't translate into a huge caloric expenditure. Most use about 150 calories.

  Just remember that miscalculations have negative consequences when coupled with other "cognitive food distortions" that give you license to eat off-limits foods. Many of my patients tell me that sports participation often makes them eat more, which ultimately undermines their diet plan. They may decide to share chocolate cake with their exercise partners after leaving the gym or the tennis court. You have to get rid of that faulty rule of thumb, "I exercise; therefore, I can eat more food!" Give up these misconceptions, or they can lead to extra inches as you exercise.

- *Don't use inability to exercise as an excuse to overeat.* Sadly enough, sometimes lack of exercise is used as a fallback position: "I don't have time to work out, so why diet?" The worst distortion I hear from women (and occasionally from men) is that exercise and dieting are inextricably linked. This variant on a perfectionism theme is common among very overweight and obese patients who may have difficulty exercising due to "weight-related" problems in their backs or knees. It is a neat rationalization; you can't exercise, so to heck with it all! Don't throw in the towel and forget about the whole arsenal of healthy interventions. Don't use your "inability to exercise" as an excuse to overeat or to defer dieting. I have patients in wheelchairs who have lost fifty to one hundred pounds. Many of my patients also continue to lose weight during periods of exercise cutbacks due to injury.

- *If you can't exercise, don't comfort yourself with extra calories.* Ultimately, gaining more weight will be anything but a comfort. Even if you don't have time for a formal exercise program, you can find forms of movement that work for you, no doubt about it. The key rules are:
- Get your doctor's approval before you start (many forms of movement can be highly aerobic).
- Start slow and work up very gradually.

Here are some good options:

- *Dance and move to music.* Most women like to dance. You may be fond of dance steps to music from periods in your life (high school or college) when you danced more often. Whether you twist, cha-cha, mambo, rumba, samba, salsa, or hip-hop, the dance moves can prove to be vital steps in weight loss. Pull out your favorite CDs, or turn on a good radio station, and spend some time dancing each day. Fifteen minutes is good enough. Plus, you'll find that moving to music does more than burn calories—it can be a mood elevator. What a great, inexpensive, essentially risk-free antidepressant. Everyone's happy on the dance floor.

  Start slowly and pick up the pace. Or follow the leader by watching exercise tapes and DVDs with dance-based exercise routines. Want company? You can always find a dance class at the local Y or sign up for ballroom dancing lessons. Just remember to work up very gradually, especially in the beginning, and have fun!
- *Partner up and go for walks.* Find someone to walk with: friend, mate, and/or child. Or take your baby outside for strolls. You get to enjoy the great outdoors. You move. You feel more energetic.

  Try walking in the morning before work, during your lunch hour, or after work, as a time to wind down. If you walk with a partner, the time will pass quickly. If no one's around, pets and earphones (iPods and other mp3 players) are great sidekicks. Just remember to keep the volume down and stay alert so that you can hear sirens or unsavory characters, and be sure to consider the safety of the area where you walk.

Make Movement Your New Mantra

Try these easy ways of working more movement into your daily life:

- *Park as far away as possible* at the mall and at work; use the stairs instead of the elevator (increase by one flight each week).
- *Use a pedometer.* This great device will get you going and keep you moving. Pedometers are inexpensive—about ten dollars. Set your sights on a goal of ten thousand steps per day, and use your pedometer to keep track. These little gadgets are invaluable aids for motivating you to burn more calories, especially if you're a woman with no time to exercise who perpetually postpones the start-up date of her exercise program.
- *Fidget as you multitask.* Move your arms and feet while you're on the phone or the Internet. How much energy you expend "at rest" is an important factor in the total number of calories you use each day in long-term weight regulation. Some researchers hypothesize that your "fidget factor" may be more important than the energy you expend during exercise. Babies who move in their cribs appear to be destined for slimmer bodies than nurserymates who lie still when swaddled. Sophisticated calorimetric devices in million-dollar clinical research centers have shown that couch potatoes can lose weight by fidgeting as they click. Tapping your toes while surfing the Net can help you lose weight.
- *Empower yourself with weight training.* Women can gain a lot from weight training, but the benefits go beyond muscle toning, osteoporosis prevention, and improved strength and coordination. Women who weight train and sculpt their bodies have higher self-esteem and a greater sense of control of their lives. Of course, we all know that women have more body fat and less lean mass than men. What's less well known is that lean mass determines resting energy expenditure—in other words, how many calories you burn during the day. So that underscores the value of a weight-training regimen. Resistance training,

weight lifting, and weight circuits are important options to tone your muscles and complement your walking program and your dance moves.

We've come a long way, baby. You can now buy sets of lower-weight weights in the one-, two-, and five-pound ranges in a drugstore or supermarket. This is a great improvement over older weight sets designed for men and bodybuilders that started at ten pounds and went up in ten-pound increments.

Use them in one hand (unless you have a speakerphone or belt clip) while you're talking on the telephone or watching TV. Keep them near your phone or television set as a reminder (but don't trip over them when you're preoccupied). If you don't see woman-friendly weights at your supermarket, you can use those sixteen-ounce soup cans you'll be buying for lunch.

- *Work out with a trainer to jump-start your program.* Studies suggest that women are more injury prone than men. A trainer is particularly important if you have Syndrome W and you're an unconditioned midlife woman who hasn't exercised for several years. A trainer can help you set up your exercise program and can

  - Demonstrate the correct method for lunges and crunches and wall-sits that seem deceptively easy in pictures
  - Prevent injury by supervising and correcting your maneuvers
  - Give coaching, feedback, and motivation
  - Serve as a role model for fitness

  But, as mentioned earlier, be sure to get your doctor's clearance for exercise first. In my own personal odyssey, working with a trainer at two transition points in my life had excellent benefits. Getting rid of upper-arm jiggle convinced me that even twice a week with a great trainer can make a great deal of difference in your level of overall fitness. It also helps motivate my patients who return year after year to chart their progress and sometimes comment on mine. Practice what you preach or you'll be a poor physician!

- *Say yes to yoga.* Last of all (and maybe it should be first of all), add yoga to your day. Yoga doesn't burn calories. But yoga's stretches and related meditation techniques are important for midlife women. The Complementary and Alternate Medicine section of the National Institutes of Health spends millions of dollars each year to demonstrate the benefits of relaxation and meditation on health and longevity.

I've seen the payoffs of yoga in some of my busiest patients, who spend as few as ten minutes a day quieting their minds and relaxing their muscles. They cite yoga as a critical aspect of their success in overcoming obesity.

The commercialization of simplicity is now big business. But you don't have to spend a lot of time or money on the right clothes and the right setting.

Ways to get your yoga fix include the following:

- Buy, download, or borrow a yoga CD or tape. You can learn the "salute to the sun" in the privacy of your own living room (before starting your day or after your children are in bed at night).
- Sign up for inexpensive adult yoga classes at a community center, YWCA, or local health club.
- Buy a how-to book or download information from the Internet.

You'll find lots of ways to add movement to your day. So forget all your old excuses. Just choose activities that you like, and keep doing them. Start with small steps and don't despair if you miss a day. Put it at the top of your priority list. Flag it in your "tasks" folder. Make up your mind, and just do it.

Chapter 23

FINALE: HINTS, HANDOUTS, AND FAQS

A Few More Tips for Living la Vida Mogul

TO HELP PEOPLE EAT BETTER AT HOME AND AT WORK, we give them all kinds of support material for losing weight permanently. My hand-outs are a work in progress that we add to all the time. We update these with suggestions from people on the Carb-Modified Diet and with tips on appealing new products that come down the supermarket pike.

The handouts are helpful because they translate all those science-y principles into simple ways to change what and when you eat. They go beyond the one-size-fits-all diet mentality, with lots of ideas for healthy food choices that don't seem like diet fare—things that I like and eat myself. They include ways to navigate at parties and how to cheat with-out straying too far. In the spirit of the color focus of the Carb-Modified Diet, the handouts are reproduced in hues of the rainbow. Color-coded and collated into packets, they virtually disappear from my desk each week. People are always asking, "Any new forms?" These handouts are the key to ensuring long-term success with the Mogul Protocol.

Staying on Top of Food

To keep handouts up to date, I regularly check out new products at the supermarket and sample the latest soups, salad dressings, and sauces. We now face a dizzying array of "lower"-carb products as food manu-facturers race to keep up with demands of low-carb dieters. Many of these products have fewer total calories and fewer added sugars, and some taste better than their higher-calorie cousins.

One of our administrators, who lost more than forty pounds and downsized from "Big Guy Clothes" to an off-the-rack size 46, told me, Diet Coke in hand, that he uses "all those forms" and particularly likes my "cheat sheet," called "Carbohydrate-Reduced Chocolates and Other Treats" (see below). He shares copies with other med-school staffers who stop by his office. He tells us he keeps the handouts close at hand because he gets more requests for copies of those than for any other forms he uses.

Carbohydrate-Reduced Chocolates and Other Treats

Although *fruits are the best way to end a meal, you'll probably want some suggestions for occasional sweets.* One caveat: please don't "overdose" on nonsugar-added supplements. Findings show that even nonsugar-based "sweets" (such as diet soda) sensitize the palate and reinforce carbohydrate cravings. So be wise and *limit these to one or two a day.*

Canfield diet soda. Use this noncaloric drink as is or as the base for a chocolate shake with no-sugar-added ice cream (Edy's or Healthy Choice).

Edy's or Healthy Choice no-sugar-added low-fat ice cream. This comes in many flavors and does contain some sugar. Measure and limit to one-half cup (one medium scoop).

Skinny Cow Silhouette bar. Here's the primo treat; it's four ounces, 110 calories, not overly sweet, and the absolute favorite of most of our patients!

Carb control ice-cream bars

Jell-O sugar-free chocolate pudding (available both as a mix or already prepared)

Aunt Gussie's no-sugar-added chocolate-chip cookies (fifty calories each and very tasty due to the large number of natural ingredients used)

Swiss Miss no-sugar-added hot chocolate/cocoa mix

Tofutti-Cuties "ice-cream" sandwiches (these are nondairy and made with soy substitutes)

Eskimo Pie bar (no-sugar-added version)

TCBY sugar-free chocolate syrup. You can use two tablespoons in skim milk or as a sundae on no-sugar ice cream.

Heavenly Desserts no-sugar-added meringues. These are virtually noncaloric, great flavored, and excellent alternatives to overly sweet nonfat meringues in tubs.

Many websites and stores have chocolate-based sugar-free (or rather "no-sugar-added") products, and these are great treats after your new eating patterns are established. But do note that I don't encourage eating candy, cookies, cakes, and so on until you have three months of weight loss going for you. Sweets can easily become a problem in the early months of the program!

The Guilt-Free Shopping Sprees: Supermarket Products 2010

1. Soups

Soups improve satiety—the feeling of fullness that signals your brain to stop eating. The list of great soups has grown dramatically. You can now find low-calorie, low-fat soups in all supermarket chains and even those stands at the gas station. Here's the latest list.

In the Frozen Food Section

Tabachnick's—These are flavorful and low in calories; some are low in sodium.

Woodstock's—Organic. Avoid high-fat choices (corn-cheese chowder)

Canned Soups

Some are high in fat and sodium. Read the labels and check the number of servings per can (one versus two). Don't worry about the few carbs you'll encounter in the mix of vegetables.

Progresso has expanded the number of vegetable, chicken, and turkey options and now has more than twenty of these in the two-hundred-calorie-per-can range. They are tasty and filling.

Campbell's Select and Healthy Choice now have a whole range of new soups.

Amy's Organic Soups, Hain, and Nature Valley have many good choices but tend to be higher in price than other brands.

Swanson's vegetable broth is by far the best-tasting broth.

Soups in a Carton

Many new choices are now available.

> Check out the soups at www.traderjoes.com. Despite the "cream" in the title, most are low in calories, low in fat, and low in sodium compared with other soups; many are eighty calories per cup.
> Imagine is widely available, and Campbell is now making soup in cartons.

2. Protein Products

Tuna and chicken—Many new ready-to-eat products are on the shelves. Available in one or two servings per package, they can be stored at home or office and added to veggies and greens for a quick and easy lunch.

Soy-based burgers, sausages, "ground meat"—Morningstar and Boca keep expanding their product line.

Hebrew National makes low-fat and even nonfat beef franks, and Empire, Perdue, and Ball Park all make chicken and turkey hot dogs. Watch the sodium; some are very high!

Low-fat chicken and turkey cold cuts (e.g., Boar's Head) are now even lower in fat and calories. (Skip those with honey, and remove all the skin.)

Egg Beaters now come in many flavored versions (e.g., Southwestern) that make great omelets and frittatas.

Kozy Shack no-sugar-added rice pudding is ninety calories per four ounces and counts as a milk serving!

3. Carbs and Condiments

Thomas now makes a whole-wheat English muffin—eighty calories, eight grams of fiber per muffin. Use half for an occasional (once-a-week) breakfast treat.

Kraft's latest low-fat mayonnaise with olive oil is low in calories and high in flavor without that artificial taste that often accompanies many low-fat versions of mayo.

What You'll Want to Know

Here are those frequently asked questions (FAQs) for an overview of the dietary program and those all-important additional details.

Q. What's unique about this diet?

It's the first dietary program that

- Lets you have "starches" (refined carbohydrates) but instructs you to eat them *later* in the day
- Mandates two (and allows up to four) servings of dietary calcium per day
- Minimizes measuring most foods—everything but fats—to make long-term weight management manageable and *easy*
- Includes a "weekly treat," normally off-limits to all dieters, with specific rules, so you don't overindulge
- Provides a long list of healthy, taste-filled foods that you already love, so you learn to give up "diets" forever!

Q. What makes it a "Carb-Modified Diet?"

Eliminating sugar, curtailing starches, and eating those starches later in the day are the cornerstones of the flexible food plan. *It's all about the timing and the quality of carbohydrates rather than total carbohydrate content.*

We know our form of dietary moderation isn't *sexy*. You're not encouraged to eat five strips of bacon for breakfast or opt for cheese cubes over cauliflower as your snack of choice. As now confirmed by many other researchers, the type and timing of those carbohydrates are critically important in diet and health. Low-glycemic-index (high-fiber) foods affect the production of important fuels in the body as well as stress hormones and appetite signals from the gut and the brain. So modifying the carbs you eat and when you eat them makes a difference in modulating hunger levels. Our simple-to-follow food exchange program provides great variety, promotes good health, and works well for everyone—but especially for people with elevated insulin levels (hyperinsulinemia).

Q. How does the Carb-Modified Diet compare with other popular low-carbohydrate diets?

It

- Exceeds the daily carb content of any and all of the popular low-carbohydrate diets out there. Depending on which foods you choose, you'll end up with about 50 percent of your total calories as carbohydrates.

- Allows three servings of whole grains or other starches (up to 300 calories total) each day after 4 p.m. (in addition to three fruits), so *you can have plenty of pasta guilt free while you lose weight!*
- Curbs excess fat *and* excludes all "added" sugars

Q. How does the diet differ from the Mediterranean diet?

The Carb-Modified Diet is a markedly *modified* Mediterranean diet. It

- Embraces *all* the fresh foods of the Mediterranean—vegetables, fish, and fruits.
- Translates concepts into specifics based on the four layers of the 4-3-2-1 pyramid. (Nutritionists agree that the Mediterranean diet needs more definition at present.)
- Advocates olive oil *but* allows other fat options that you can tailor to your own tastes *and* restricts these to two servings (200–250 calories per day) to keep calories down. (Fats are densely caloric and must be watched for weight loss.)
- Limits nuts. At ten nuts (one-half ounce) for one hundred calories and eight hundred calories for the typical "snack-size" serving you'll find on the shelves and at the candy counter, nuts can spell trouble for dieters who overindulge.

Q. Why does it matter what time of day I eat my three daily starches?

Postponing starches until later in the day is the key component of our diet. It dates back to the diet I devised at Barnard College twenty-five years ago. The concept is continually reinforced by the comments of patient after patient, including women and men of all ages from our clinical practice, affiliated clinic, and research studies. Virtually all report a surge in hunger in the late morning or early afternoon when they have those carbs at breakfast (whether it's low-fat muffins or high-fiber cereal) that just doesn't occur when the first meal of the day is limited to protein. Avoiding added sugars and starches early in the morning diminishes your desire for a doughnut before lunch. Test the rules yourself and see. You'll find that you're less hungry and less tired in the late morning when you give up the breakfast granola.

Q. Why can't I have a high-fiber cereal or oatmeal for breakfast?

If you have Syndrome W, you have an elevated insulin response curve, which means that even high-fiber breakfast food will trigger an insulin response. If you really miss your oatmeal or need fiber for regularity, eat a bowl of oatmeal as your four o'clock snack. (Just make sure you don't choose instant oats.) Once-a-week oatmeal for breakfast also works, but *for long-term weight maintenance, you need to find other foods to eat and reduce your reliance on oatmeal and other high-fiber, whole-grain breakfast foods.* This can be a major stumbling block for some of my patients until they notice that their favorite high-fiber breakfast cereal makes a difference—they don't feel as well as when they eat one of the other breakfast options. They also notice that they're a lot hungrier on days when they indulge in those old favorites. I'm an empiricist (driven by observation), so I encourage you to go ahead, experiment, and see for yourself. (Just try not to venture too far from camp.)

Q. What about a sandwich on low-calorie, high-grain fiber bread for lunch?

For maximal success, you have to decrease starches at both lunch and breakfast. While whole-grain breads are certainly better than breads made from overprocessed wheat flours, they're still carbohydrates and cause a spike in insulin levels. The key of the Carb-Modified Diet regimen is postponing starches until later in the day. *Soup and salad work time and again for my patients. This is the critical dietary change that's necessary for your long-term success.* Have your main meal at lunch instead of dinner if you prefer. Just keep starches off your plate and pile it with low-fat protein and lots of vegetables. Sample the bounty of great soups, protein-rich salads, and vegetable entrées.

Not sure about this? See how many people nod off during those afternoon meetings. Check out what the nappers ate for lunch. Truth is, it's easy to wind up supersluggish an hour after eating one of those otherwise healthy pita wraps. So get off the sandwich kick altogether, and move on to healthier eating. You'll have much less downtime in the afternoon.

Q. Do I have to do all that measuring and weighing to make this work?

No. You really don't have to worry about an extra cup of string beans or strawberries or an extra ounce or two of skinned chicken breast. We like to keep things simple. So we suggest you focus mainly on measuring fats. Fats are calorically dense, so a few extra tablespoons of olive oil can spell trouble and add lots of extra unintended calories if you're not careful. Get a good set of measuring spoons to measure oil, butter, and mayo and a postage scale to weigh cheese or divide a preweighed package of low-fat cheese into one-ounce sections or slices. Avoid the pain of the diet plateau of one patient of mine, who reported that she ate only chicken breasts and salad and later disclosed (after lots of questions) that she "just sprinkled a little olive oil" from the bottle onto the greens! Remember, other calorically dense foods—candies, cakes, cookies, cereals (the four *C*s)—are off limits from the get-go. Also learn the visual cues for eyeballing portion sizes of pasta and low-fat proteins. A typical protein serving is the size of a deck of cards, and a serving of ice cream is a scoop size that's midway between a golf ball and a tennis ball.

Q. What about the sugar in diet dressings? What labels do I really have to read?

First, read the "total caloric content" per serving (usually one to two tablespoons or one ounce) on the label. If it's thirty-five calories or less and you typically use one serving on your salad, you don't need to go any further. Reading labels can definitely steer you to the right products. But as a general rule for dressings or sauces in the forty- to fifty-calorie-per-serving range, see where sugar is listed under "ingredients." If it's not in the first three ingredients listed, you're fine. Remember, too, that "high-fructose corn syrup" is sugar. Any condiment that's more than fifty calories per one-ounce serving is calorically dense and undesirable.

Q. Wouldn't I be better off if I didn't eat the weekly treat?

When you're revising your eating plan "for life," you need to be realistic. Regardless of great progress on all fronts, you can be sure that you're eventually going to want a slice of birthday cake, or Aunt Polly's pumpkin pie at Thanksgiving, or Mocho-Choco Madness on Saturday night. Part of long-term dietary change is making room for treats. Remember, *dietary deprivation can lead to disaster; so it's important to find a way to add some forbidden fruit to your daily fruits. Figure on a 300–350 calorie serving, and follow the rules.* Plan your treat and enjoy it guilt free, preferably in the company of others. If you'd rather eat your treat at home, alone, buy a portion-size serving, not a whole cake, or a small brownie or cupcake. Have a small sundae or wedge of pie, not a banana split or a diner-size chunk of cheesecake. Make sure your weekly treat doesn't morph into a daily treat. And keep any "trigger foods"—those temptations that you can't control—completely off the list. Otherwise, indulge.

Q. What about protein bars for a snack or an "emergency" situation?

Let me say it once and for all, loud and clear, double-bold-highlighted, exclamation point—ban the bars! Those innocent-looking "healthy" treats may not have any sugar, carbs, or fat, but they are among the most calorically dense protein foods around. They have no place in your cupboard or your car.

Look at their drawbacks:

- Poor substitutes for meals
- Rarely tasty
- Completely processed protein products and sugar substitutes
- Gram for gram, expensive

They are today's *grand illusion* for healthy eating. At least a Pop-Tart doesn't profess to be healthy. Eat an orange or an apple, a hard-boiled egg, or a single package (thirty-five to one hundred calories) one-ounce serving of low-fat cheese, like Laughing Cow light or Bonbel. The only bar that belongs in your list of diet staples is the no-sugar-added ice-cream bar. Buy these and bypass all the others.

Q. I really don't have time for breakfast, so what should I do?

You don't have to have breakfast food for breakfast. If, like most of my patients, you have absolutely no time for a sit-down meal, don't worry. There are lots of legal options. At the top of my list is always a low-fat (skim) latte (decaf or regular). This drink is a great protein-rich staple of my diet and tastier than many breakfast options. Lattes are an excellent source of calcium and vitamin D, nutrients important in preserving bone health for midlife women (and for building bone in younger women). If you are lactose intolerant, buy a soy-milk-based version, widely available in coffee shops. Don't like coffee? Do a chai latte using chai tea bags (never the mixes) steeped in hot milk.

The protein staves off hunger for hours. Plus, drinking a latte when you're pressed for time helps you avoid eating-on-the-run behaviors that are often detrimental to long-term behavior change. Check out the recipe for that morning mug (chapter 21) and other low-carb breakfast options (chapter 16) for more suggestions.

Q. Can I postpone my dessert at dinner until later in the evening?

Definitely! That's a great strategy if your "decompress" time includes an hour or two in front of the TV or catching up with the news near the kitchen. Since food cues on TV and in newspapers and magazines make us want to eat all night, it's a good idea to set aside time about an hour before bedtime to enjoy a treat—a bar (Skinny Cow, Healthy Choice, or Weight Watchers), or a scoop of no-sugar-added Edy's ice cream, or low-fat yogurt with a cup of berries. If you really can eat just one, this is a good time for a half-ounce to one-ounce cookie or biscotti (maximum of 120 calories) with a cup of herbal tea or warm milk (skim or 2 percent). Relax and enjoy. Establish new evening routines and replace the old to eliminate barriers and create bridges to long-term success.

Q. What's the best way to handle eating out, fast food, travel, and parties?

Be prepared and plan ahead. The Carb-Modified Diet has extensive choices, which means few eateries are off-limits. Patients report that's their favorite thing about our program. Three daily starches and that weekly treat allow you to be part of the party painlessly. And metformin adds that extra measure of control that lets you live in and enjoy the real world of food without major transgressions. Enjoy the confidence and the comfort level that come with using this combination regimen. And have fun everywhere you go.

Q. Does the program work for people who don't have Syndrome W or insulin resistance?

Absolutely!

Part V

DELICIOUS RECIPES
FROM GREAT CHEFS

About the Recipes

HERE ARE SOME OF MY FAVORITE RECIPES for soups, salads, side dishes, fish, fowl, and not-so-forbidden fruits from award-winning chefs and favorite food shops from Chappaqua, New York, and Vail, Colorado, plus just a few from the author. They all they have amazing flavor and infinite variations that are all low in fat, low in calories, and healthy. The recipes on these pages range from simple to complex. Many can be prepared and on the table in under thirty minutes or frozen in advance and reheated. A few entrées and desserts are special-occasion fare that's not meant for frenzied weeknight dinners.

You won't find the customary caloric analyses included with the recipes, and that's because such analyses can be misleading, particularly in the case of meat or fish dishes, where caloric content varies significantly, depending on fat content. "Lean" ground turkey or beef can vary dramatically from meat counter to meat counter and state to state and can contain 5 percent or even 15 percent fat. Age, cut, variety, and environmental waters all influence the fat content of salmon and other healthy "fatty" fishes. The grade and degree of doneness determines the fat content and, ultimately, the calorie count of beef. Also, butter from France has a higher content of fat (and a lower content of water) than U.S. butter. Even the caloric content of fruit can vary somewhat, depending on variety and ripeness.

The goal of the dietary directives in this book is lifestyle change through broad new culinary initiatives, with expanded food choices based on fresh and flavorful vegetables, fruits, and low-fat protein in moderate portions. So have fun in the kitchen, and try to focus on the big picture.

SOUPS

Generic Green Soup
Harriette Mogul

Orange Soup
Harriette Mogul

Intense Asparagus Soup with Truffle Oil
Steve Topple

Vegetarian Black Bean Soup
Giona Stanco

Roasted Cauliflower Soup
Giona Stanco

Chicken Vegetable Soup
Brian Peck

Burgundy Eggplant Soup
Peter Milette

Gazpacho with Dungeness Crab and Guacamole
Paul Ferzacca

Tomato Basil Soup
Giona Stanco

Yellow Tomato Soup
Mark Kramer

Generic Green Soup

This soup has an infinite number of variations, depending on which vegetables, stock, herbs, and seasonings you choose. You can serve it cold or hot, with a dollop (two tablespoons or so) of yogurt or low-fat sour cream, or crème fraîche and a sprinkling of fresh herbs. Dill, parsley, chives, and coriander all work well, but you can get fancier and use tarragon, thyme, French basil, or any of the varieties of herbs from your garden or supermarket produce aisles. You can puree it in a blender and make it silky smooth so that it tastes like a cream soup sans cream, or serve it with a little more texture after fewer turns in the food processor. My own personal favorite is a mix; I puree most of the contents of the pot and add the rest, which I've kept a bit coarser.

Here are my directions and a recipe for the soup, suitable for additional varieties from the color spectrum. Although you do not have to use these exact measurements, it's important to use the same proportions.

YIELD: 6 QUARTS (24 1-CUP SERVINGS)

Ingredients

3 large Spanish or Bermuda onions (about 1 pound each), coarsely chopped, or 2 large onions and 6 leeks, white parts only, well rinsed, halved, and cut into 1-inch lengths

3 tablespoons extra-virgin olive oil

3 large bunches broccoli or 3 pounds zucchini

1 large Yukon Gold or Red Bliss potato, scrubbed (not peeled), halved, cut in ½-inch slices

8–10 cups quality canned vegetable or chicken stock (you may substitute 8–10 cups water plus 10 individual-serving packages of consommé powder or bouillon cubes)

6–8 large sprigs fresh dill or Italian parsley (roots removed) or ¼ cup mixed chopped fresh herbs or 4 tablespoons dried dill weed or fines herbes

Freshly ground black pepper to taste

1. Add onions and olive oil to 8-quart stockpot and mix well. Cover and place over low heat for 10 minutes until onions are translucent but not brown.

2. Remove florets from the broccoli and set aside. Trim coarse outer fiber from the outside of the broccoli stalks and cut into 1-inch chunks. If you are using zucchini, slice into ½-inch rounds after removing the stem and bottom tip.

3. Remove pot from stove. Add chunked vegetables, potato slices, and broccoli florets (in that order).
4. Cover the vegetables with the stock.
5. Bring to a gentle boil, then turn down heat and simmer for 25 minutes, uncovered.
6. Add fresh herbs and cook an additional 5 minutes until the vegetables are completely cooked.
7. Cool completely.
8. Using a soup ladle, puree in blender or food processor in batches to desired consistency. Do not fill blender or food processor more than three-fourths full.
9. Season to taste with fresh pepper or other spices as suggested and mix well.
10. Freeze in 1-quart containers.

Variations

1. Mixed Green Soup: Substitute 2 pounds fresh or frozen peas for 1 or 2 of the broccoli heads.
2. Asparagus Soup: Substitute 3 large bunches of asparagus for the broccoli. Snap off the ends of the asparagus and discard (if you know how) or cut off the bottom half-inch of each stalk. Puree to a fine consistency or you will end up with a lot of fiber that eludes the blade of the food processor.
3. Spinach or Sorrel Soup: Use either 6 bunches of fresh spinach or sorrel that have been well rinsed (remove any coarse stems). Add an additional potato. You can substitute a bunch of fresh tarragon (stems removed) or 1 tablespoon dried tarragon for the dill.

Orange Soup

This is the soup I usually serve in fall and winter. It is a sweet, hearty soup that qualifies well as comfort food. I usually make it with carrots or a mixture of winter squashes (see variations below) and sometimes add parsnips for a wonderful nutty flavor. Add a cored, peeled, quartered apple in the last fifteen minutes, or substitute one cup of apple cider for a cup of the stock for additional sweetness. Despite the rich taste, orange soup is low in calories. When I serve this soup in seasons other than fall/winter, I typically add yogurt and curry and garnish the dollop of low-fat sour cream or crème fraîche with a few raisins or a tablespoon per serving of chopped pistachio or hazelnuts (or slivered or diced almonds). I prefer this soup a bit more velvety than my green soup and recommend that you puree it in a blender. It's best made with fresh, small carrots that you buy in bunches with the greens still attached, but anything works, even the peeled smaller carrots available year-round in supermarkets. Just avoid overly large, overly dried carrots with a diameter of two inches or more.

YIELD: 4 QUARTS (16 1-CUP SERVINGS)

Ingredients

3 large Spanish or Bermuda onions (about 1 pound each), coarsely chopped, or 2 large onions and 6 leeks, white parts only, well rinsed, halved lengthwise and cut into 1-inch pieces

2 tablespoons extra-virgin olive oil

5 bunches (about 1 pound each, or 8 cups) carrots, peeled and cut in half-inch slices (see hint below on how to cut carrots into similar sizes)

10–12 cups quality canned vegetable or chicken stock (or 10 cups water plus 10 individual-serving packages of consommé powder or bouillon cubes)

2 walnut-size pieces fresh ginger, peeled, chopped finely, or 2 tablespoons quality curry powder

Freshly ground pepper (using white, black, or a mixture of peppercorns) to taste

2 cups low-fat yogurt or 1 cup low-fat half-and-half

1. Add the onions and olive oil to a 6-quart stockpot and mix well. Cover and place over low heat for 10 minutes until the onions are translucent but not brown.

2. In the meantime, cut carrots as described.

3. Remove pot from stove and add chunked vegetables.
4. Cover the vegetables with the stock.
5. Bring to a gentle boil, then turn down heat, and simmer for 25–30 minutes, uncovered, until the vegetables are completely cooked.
6. Turn off heat and add ginger or curry.
7. Cool *completely*.
8. Using a soup ladle, puree in blender in batches to desired consistency.
9. Season to taste with fresh pepper and mix well.
10. To serve, reheat. Remove from stove and blend in yogurt (if desired). Garnish and enjoy.
11. Freeze in 1-quart containers (without yogurt).

Hint: To guarantee uniform cooking, keep the carrot slices thinner (e.g., ½ inch at the widest width) and cut them progressively wider toward the tip of the carrot.

Variations

1. Substitute any of the following for half of the carrots: parsnips, butternut squash, or any winter squash that is peeled, seeded, and cut in 1-inch cubes.
2. For an elegant dinner party, substitute low-fat half-and-half for the yogurt and mix well. (Add prior to heating or freezing.) Garnish each serving with quartered or coarsely chopped walnuts that have been warmed in a 350°F oven for 5 minutes.
3. For a summer patio presentation, serve chilled in clear glass mugs with a dollop of yogurt, crème fraîche, or low-fat sour cream and a garnish of fresh chives, dill, mint, or chervil.

Intense Asparagus Soup with Truffle Oil

YIELD: 6 SERVINGS

Ingredients

2 shallots, peeled and finely sliced

1 stick celery, washed and sliced thin

4 cloves garlic, chopped or crushed

2 large potatoes, peeled and diced

¼ cup oil

3 bunches asparagus

2 cups vegetable stock (you can use cubes from the supermarket)

2 cups spinach, washed

Salt and pepper to taste

1 ounce white truffle oil (available at most good supermarkets)

1. In a large pot, sauté the shallots, celery, garlic, and potatoes in a small amount of oil.
2. Chop the bunches of asparagus; keep the tops for a garnish. Chop three-fourths of the remaining asparagus spears very small so that they cook evenly. Add to the pot to cook. Continue cooking for 10 minutes.
3. Add vegetable stock over the ingredients in the pot, and simmer for 35 minutes. Just before taking the soup off, add spinach. (This helps keep it green.)
4. Puree, using a stick blender or a drink blender; be careful not to fill the drink blender too much.
5. Strain the soup, using a fine strainer. Season the soup, and check the consistency. Use a little more water if you need to.
6. In a small saucepan, boil some water with a little salt. Add the tops of the asparagus; drain and serve in the soup.
7. Pour the soup into serving bowls. Garnish with the tops of asparagus and a little drizzle of truffle oil.

Vegetarian Black Bean Soup

Ingredients

2 cups dried black beans

2 tablespoons olive oil

1 medium yellow onion, diced

1 stalk celery, chopped

1 carrot, diced

2 plum tomatoes, peeled and roughly chopped

3 cloves garlic, chopped

2 tablespoons flat-leaf parsley

1 tablespoon dried sage

1 bay leaf

½ teaspoon ground cumin

½ teaspoon chili powder

1½ teaspoons salt

Freshly ground black pepper to taste

2 quarts low-sodium vegetable stock (homemade or store-bought) or water

1. In a glass or stainless-steel bowl, soak beans overnight in cool water to cover in the refrigerator. Drain before cooking. Do not reserve soaking water.
2. To a large saucepan heated over medium heat, add olive oil. Heat oil briefly; add onion, celery, and carrot.
3. Toss for a minute; add tomatoes, garlic, herbs, and spices. Toss for an additional minute.
4. Add the beans, turning and toasting for 90 seconds—this will provide soup with its unique nutty flavor.
5. To the pan, add 2 quarts of hot vegetable stock or water (you don't want to slow the cooking); cover, bring to boil, uncover, and simmer for 2 hours.
6. If the soup requires additional liquid, add 1–2 cups hot water. When beans reach semisoft consistency, adjust for seasoning with salt and pepper. Serve hot.

Roasted Cauliflower Soup

Ingredients

1 large head fresh cauliflower, cut into eighths—or whatever size will fit comfortably and in a single layer on a stainless-steel sheet pan (or cookie sheet)

1 medium yellow onion, roughly cut

1 stalk celery, chopped

1 medium carrot, chopped

3 cloves fresh garlic, flattened

2 quarts water (keep 2 quarts heated, but start with 1 quart, adding more if needed; using stock in this recipe results in overly dark soup)

3 tablespoons olive oil

Salt and pepper to taste

2 tablespoons fresh flat-leaf parsley

2 tablespoons fresh sage, roughly chopped

1. Preheat oven to 425°F.
2. Place cauliflower, onion, celery, carrot, and garlic onto sheet pan. Season with salt and pepper. Drizzle with 2 tablespoons olive oil. Place on rack in middle of oven.
3. Roast for approximately 20 minutes—or until veggies begin to caramelize. Remove from oven.
4. In a medium-size saucepan over medium heat, pour remaining 1 tablespoon olive oil. Heat 1 minute.
5. Add all of the roasted veggies and enough water to cover. Bring to a soft boil. Add parsley and sage.
6. Cover pan, lower heat to medium, and let simmer 30 minutes.
7. Adjust for seasoning.
8. Remove pan from stove. Blend with hand blender. Serve hot.

Chicken Vegetable Soup

YIELD: 4 SERVINGS

Ingredients

4 ounces chopped carrots

4 ounces chopped celery

4 ounces chopped onion

1 teaspoon garlic

1 cup plum tomatoes (canned), chopped

4 cups chicken broth

1 cheesecloth sachet. Place all spices in cheesecloth, tie with string:

1 teaspoon peppercorns

½ teaspoon dried oregano

½ teaspoon dried basil

2 bay leaves

½ pound chicken breasts

1 cup fresh spinach, shredded

4 teaspoons grated chèvre

1. Sauté carrots for 2 minutes.
2. Add celery and onions and sauté until translucent.
3. Add garlic, tomatoes, chicken broth, and sachet, and cook for 20 minutes.
4. Poach chicken breasts until fully cooked.
5. Chop chicken into small pieces and add to soup.
6. Squeeze sachet with tongs into soup; remove sachet.
7. Add shredded spinach and cheese.
8. Serve with warm bread or sprinkle with croutons.

Burgundy Eggplant Soup

Ingredients

2 eggplants

¼ cup olive oil

2 cups burgundy wine

1 tablespoon garlic, minced

1 tablespoon shallots, minced

4 cups chicken stock

2 tablespoons chopped rosemary

Salt and pepper to taste

¼ cup grated parmesan cheese

1. Preheat oven to 400°F.
2. Peel eggplants and cut in half lengthwise.
3. Coat eggplants with olive oil and roast in oven 30 minutes.
4. Puree roasted eggplants in food processor.
5. In heavy 2-quart saucepan, reduce wine by half, with garlic and shallots.
6. Add chicken stock and pureed eggplant.
7. Season with rosemary, salt, and pepper. Simmer for 20 minutes. Top each serving with parmesan.

Gazpacho with Dungeness Crab and Guacamole

YIELD: 4 SERVINGS

Gazpacho Ingredients

2½ pounds vine-ripened tomatoes, chopped

1 medium green bell pepper, chopped

1 medium red bell pepper, chopped

1 small red onion, chopped

2 cucumbers, peeled, seeded, and chopped

1 serrano chile

2 garlic cloves

1 tablespoon extra-virgin olive oil

1 cup tomato juice

3 tablespoons sherry vinegar (or to taste)

Salt to taste

Ground white pepper to taste

1. In a blender, puree tomatoes, green pepper, red pepper, red onion, cucumbers, serrano chile, garlic, olive oil, and tomato juice.
2. Once completely pureed, add a little sherry vinegar, salt, and ground white pepper to taste.
3. Chill completely, preferably overnight.
4. You can thin the soup with more tomato juice or ice water if necessary.

Crab Guacamole Ingredients

2 avocados, skinned, pits removed, diced into ½-inch pieces

½ small red onion, diced, or 2 tablespoons

1 roma tomato, diced into ¼-inch pieces

1 clove garlic, minced

1 tablespoon cilantro, chopped

Juice of ½ small lime

¼ pound Dungeness crab, cleaned of any shell

Salt to taste

Ground white pepper to taste

1. In a bowl, combine avocados, red onion, tomato, garlic, cilantro, lime juice, and crab.
2. Mix well. Season with salt and ground white pepper.
3. Use this mixture to garnish gazpacho soup.

Tomato Basil Soup

YIELD: 4 SERVINGS

Ingredients

2 tablespoons olive oil

1 medium yellow onion, chopped

1 medium carrot, finely chopped

1 stalk celery, cleaned and chopped

28-ounce can peeled plum tomatoes
  or San Marzano tomatoes (with
  juices), roughly chopped

¼ cup chopped fresh basil
  (leaves only)

1 teaspoon sugar
  (or sugar substitute)

Salt and pepper to taste

½ cup whole milk
  (or fat-free milk)

1. In a medium heavy-bottom saucepan, over medium heat, add olive oil. Let oil warm for almost a minute; add onion, carrot, and celery. Sauté, but do not brown, about 90 seconds over medium heat.
2. Add tomatoes, basil, sugar, salt, and pepper. Bring to soft boil. Lower heat to medium. Let cook for 20 minutes.
3. In cooking pan, blend with a hand blender.
4. Return to heat, add milk. Simmer (don't boil) for 2 minutes. Adjust seasonings.
5. Serve hot, at room temperature, or chilled. Great accompanied by homemade crostini!

Yellow Tomato Soup

YIELD: 4 SERVINGS

Ingredients

2 tablespoons extra-virgin olive oil
1 yellow onion, peeled and chopped
3 stalks celery, chopped
2 carrots, chopped
10 medium yellow tomatoes, stems
    removed, quartered

4 garlic cloves, chopped
1 quart chicken stock
Pinch saffron
Salt and freshly ground black pepper
    to taste

1. In a large, heavy-bottom saucepan, heat olive oil to medium heat.
2. Add onion, celery, and carrots. Cook until vegetables are slightly soft and have a very slight golden color, about 6–8 minutes.
3. Add tomatoes, garlic, chicken stock, and saffron.
4. Season lightly with salt and pepper.
5. Cover and reduce heat to low. Stir occasionally.
6. When tomatoes, onions, and garlic are soft (about 30 minutes), remove from heat and let cool until the mixture is cool enough to handle. Puree in a blender or food processor.
7. Pour through a mesh strainer, pushing pulp through with the back of a wooden spoon. Discard seeds, peels, and fibers left in the strainer. Soup will be delicate and smooth.
8. Season to taste with more salt and pepper.
9. Serve hot or chilled.

SALADS

Asian Chicken Salad
Philip Callaci

Cajun Chicken Salad
Brian Peck

Chicken Raspberry Waldorf Salad
Brian Peck

Chicken or Turkey Salad with Fruit and Nuts
Harriette Mogul

California Coleslaw
Philip Callaci

Confetti Corn and Bean Salad
Philip Callaci

Vietnamese Shrimp Salad with Yuzu Dressing
Paul Ferzacca

Reduced-Fat Tuna Salad with Apples and Cranberries
Philip Callaci

Spa Tuna Salad
Mark Kramer

Smoked Trout Salad
Fred Mogul

Wildflower Waldorf Salad
Steve Topple

Asian Chicken Salad

Ingredients

16 ounces boneless chicken cutlets

8 ounces sesame oil

2 red Holland peppers

1 yellow Holland pepper

1 head savoy cabbage

3 cloves garlic

4 ounces teriyaki sauce

2 teaspoons powdered ginger

4 ounces honey (or Splenda)

1 teaspoon paprika

1. Brush chicken with 1 to 2 ounces of sesame oil (as needed) and grill to an internal temperature of 165°F (as recorded on an instant-read thermometer inserted into the thickest part of the chicken breast). Cool.
2. Julienne all peppers and savoy cabbage and place in large mixing bowl.
3. Julienne chicken when cool and add to pepper-cabbage mixture.
4. Make dressing as follows: Combine garlic, teriyaki sauce, powdered ginger, honey, and paprika in blender or food processor; blend well. With machine running, slowly add remaining sesame oil until fully emulsified.
5. Pour dressing on chicken mixture and serve.

Cajun Chicken Salad

Ingredients

1 teaspoon fresh garlic, minced
1 teaspoon onion powder
1 teaspoon paprika
1 teaspoon dried oregano
1 teaspoon white pepper
1 teaspoon crushed red pepper

1 teaspoon cayenne
1 teaspoon salt
4 6-ounce to 8-ounce chicken cutlets
Vegetable oil spray
Mixed greens
Ranch dressing

1. Combine garlic, onion powder, paprika, oregano, white pepper, red pepper, cayenne, and salt in a shallow bowl, and mix completely.
2. Dust both sides of chicken cutlets with Cajun spice mixture.
3. Spray dusted cutlets with vegetable oil.
4. Grill until done, approximately 4 minutes each side until no longer pink.
5. Cut chicken into ½-inch strips.
6. Serve on top of mixed greens with a side of ranch dressing.

Chicken Raspberry Waldorf Salad

Raspberry Vinaigrette Ingredients

¼ cup raspberry vinegar

2 tablespoons Dijon mustard

2 tablespoons honey

1 tablespoon chopped shallots

1 cup soy or olive oil

1. Mix all ingredients in blender until oil and vinegar are incorporated.
2. Set aside while you prepare the salad.

Waldorf Salad Ingredients

Salt and pepper to taste

4 chicken breasts

Olive oil

1 cup walnuts

Mixed baby greens

2 Granny Smith apples, peeled and sliced in wedges

1 pint raspberries

3 ounces goat cheese, crumbled

1. Salt and pepper the chicken breasts. Lightly brush with olive oil and cook on grill for 4 minutes on each side, or until no longer pink and grill marks appear.
2. Toast the walnuts for 10 minutes in a 300°F oven.
3. Slice the grilled chicken into ½-inch strips.
4. To assemble the salad, in a large bowl, toss baby greens with prepared vinaigrette and walnuts.
5. Finish by garnishing with grilled chicken, apples, raspberries, and goat cheese.

Chicken or Turkey Salad with Fruit and Nuts

YIELD: 4 SERVINGS

Ingredients

2 cups cooked turkey or chicken breasts, cubed

½ cup coarsely chopped walnuts (toast walnut halves for 10 minutes in a 300°F oven, and cool prior to chopping)

½ cup minced celery

½ cup raisins, currants, or dried apricots (scissor into ¼-inch dice)

½ cup reduced-fat mayonnaise (preferably Hellmann's or Kraft)

½ cup light sour cream

¼ cup Dijon mustard

2 tablespoons fresh lemon juice

1–2 tablespoons curry powder to taste (optional)

Salt and pepper to taste

1. In large mixing bowl, combine chicken or turkey, walnuts, celery, and dried fruits.
2. Combine remaining ingredients in a 2-cup Pyrex measuring cup or small bowl. Mix well and season to taste.
3. Pour dressing over chicken mixture.
4. Refrigerate for several hours prior to serving so that chicken will absorb the dressing. Garnish with additional chopped nuts or dried fruits as desired.

California Coleslaw

YIELD: 6 SERVINGS

Ingredients

1 head red cabbage, shredded

16 ounces shredded carrots

16 ounces zucchini, shredded in a food processor

8 ounces dried cranberries

4 ounces currants

4 ounces red wine vinegar

12 tablespoons Splenda

6 ounces olive or canola oil

1. Add cabbage, carrots, zucchini, dried cranberries, and currants to a large mixing bowl and mix well.
2. Mix vinegar and Splenda in a blender or food processor; mix well.
3. Slowly add oil to vinegar/Splenda mixture until fully emulsified.
4. Pour dressing on cabbage mixture, mix well, and serve.

Confetti Corn and Bean Salad

Ingredients

16 ounces frozen peas

16 ounces frozen corn

16-ounce can black beans, well rinsed
    and drained

1 red Holland pepper

2 cloves garlic

1 teaspoon Cajun or fajita spice mix

4 ounces olive oil

1 tablespoon fresh lemon juice

1. Mix peas and corn in large strainer and defrost under running water; place in large mixing bowl.
2. Add beans to pea and corn mixture.
3. Dice red pepper and add to mixture.
4. Finely mince garlic and add to mixture.
5. Add all other ingredients and mix well.

Note: Add salt and pepper to taste. The beans suck up the salt, so you may need to add more than you think. This salad tastes better the second day.

Vietnamese Shrimp Salad
with Yuzu Dressing

YIELD: 8 SERVINGS

Yuzu Dressing Ingredients

½ stalk lemongrass

8 ounces water

2 ounces Yuzu citrus juice
(or 1 ounce orange juice and
1 ounce lemon juice)

3 ounces sugar or Splenda

2 ounces fish sauce

¼ teaspoon Thai crushed chilies
or bird's eye chilies

½ teaspoon salt

Juice from ½ fresh lime

1. Cut lemongrass into 2-inch pieces, and combine with 8 ounces water; bring to a simmer and steep to make a lemongrass tea.
2. Chill and reserve; you need only 3 ounces lemongrass tea for the dressing.
3. In a large stainless-steel bowl, combine 3 ounces lemongrass tea, Yuzu citrus juice, sugar, fish sauce, Thai crushed chilies, salt, and lime juice.
4. Stir dressing until sugar is dissolved, and keep refrigerated until needed.

Shrimp Salad Ingredients

1 cup cabbage

¼ cup carrots, chopped

1 cup English cucumber

2 tablespoons fresh mint

2 tablespoons cilantro, minced

2 tablespoons peanuts, dry roasted

16 ounces cooked shrimp (41–50)

1 head butter lettuce

1. Cut the cabbage into matchstick-size pieces and place in large bowl.
2. Cut the carrot into matchstick-size pieces and place in bowl with cabbage.
3. Peel the cucumber and cut into small dice; place in bowl with cabbage.
4. Cut the mint into julienne and add to cabbage bowl.
5. Rough-chop the cilantro and add to cabbage bowl.
6. Chop the peanuts into small pieces and add to cabbage bowl.
7. Rough-chop the shrimp and add to cabbage bowl.
8. Tear butter lettuce into bite-size pieces and add to cabbage bowl.
9. Add Yuzu Dressing to cabbage bowl. Toss to dress all ingredients. Adjust seasoning to taste.

Reduced-Fat Tuna Salad
with Apples and Cranberries

YIELD: 4 SERVINGS

Ingredients

16-ounce can chunked white tuna
packed in water (do not substitute
"lite" tuna)

2 Fuji apples

2 tablespoons lemon juice

8 ounces dried cranberries

Salt and pepper to taste

8–16 ounces low-fat or reduced-fat
high-quality mayonnaise

1. Thoroughly drain tuna and place in large mixing bowl.
2. Peel and core apples; dice, sprinkle with lemon juice, and add
   to tuna.
3. Add cranberries, salt, pepper, and 8 ounces of mayo and mix
   thoroughly.
4. Add additional mayo, depending on how wet or dry you like tuna.

Spa Tuna Salad

YIELD: 4 SERVINGS

Ingredients

2 8-ounce cans albacore tuna packed
in water

6 radishes, thinly sliced

2 celery ribs, finely diced

1 tomato, seeds removed, diced

1 cup radicchio, shredded

¼ cup red onion, finely minced

2 tablespoons fresh lemon juice

1 tablespoon Dijon mustard

Salt and pepper to taste

Extra-virgin olive oil (optional)

1. Combine drained tuna with vegetables.
2. Whisk lemon juice into mustard, and toss with tuna mixture.
3. Season with salt and pepper. Drizzle with extra-virgin olive oil if
   desired.

Smoked Trout Salad

YIELD: 4 SERVINGS

Ingredients

1 pound smoked trout fillets, skin
   removed

½ cup ricotta cheese

1 large shallot or 2 scallions, minced

2 tablespoons fresh lime juice

2 tablespoons white horseradish

Salt and white pepper to taste

Freshly chopped chives

1. Coarsely flake trout, taking care to remove any fine bones. Put in mixing bowl.
2. Combine remaining ingredients (except chives) in bowl of food processor (or blender) and pulse until well blended.
3. Pour dressing over trout.
4. Garnish with chopped chives.

Wildflower Waldorf Salad

Ingredients

3 large Fuji apples

Juice of 1 lemon

1 teaspoon cinnamon

2 ounces brown sugar

½ cup sherry vinegar

1½ cups blended oil

Salt and pepper to taste

½ cup toasted walnuts

10 ounces mixed greens

½ cup seedless red grapes

1. Cut each apple into 8 pieces. Remove seeds and place on a baking tray.
2. Sprinkle lemon juice over apples to prevent discoloration.
3. Sprinkle cinnamon and brown sugar evenly over apples.
4. Bake in an oven at 250°F for 2 hours, until apples begin to dry a little and turn golden brown.
5. In drink blender, add sherry vinegar, blended oil seasoned with salt and pepper, and ¼ cup walnuts.
6. Puree until smooth and emulsified.
7. Toss mixed greens in a small amount of the dressing, add salt and pepper, and lay on the plate in the middle.
8. On the plate, place 6 of the apple pieces around the greens; sprinkle a few of the walnuts around and a little more of the sherry walnut dressing. Spoon the grapes around and serve.

FISH AND SEAFOOD

Mustard Horseradish-Crusted Arctic Char or Halibut
John Everin and Joe Di Mauro

Panko-Crusted Sea Bass with Tomato Provençal Sauce
Paul Ferzacca

Olive-Coated Bass with Tomato Herb Vinaigrette
Peter Milette

Wildflower Crab Cake with Vanilla-Mango Chutney
and Lemon Thyme Vinaigrette
Steve Topple

Pan-Seared John Dory with Melted Leeks and Vanilla Sauce
Steve Topple

Mussels Fra Diavolo
Brian Peck

Pistachio-Crusted Salmon
John Everin and Joe Di Mauro

Scallion-Potato-Crusted Salmon
John Everin and Joe Di Mauro

Hibachi Salmon with Soy and Sesame Glaze
Brian Peck

Seared Scallops with Pomegranate Vinaigrette
Paul Ferzacca

Salmon Cakes, Many Ways
Harriette Mogul

The fish recipes reflect the "mix and match" concept of modular cooking that I focus on in this book: a basic set of techniques to help you build your own favorite fish recipe collection. The sauces can be used interchangeably with almost any of the fishes, and the flavorful vinaigrettes and salsas can also dress greens, vegetables, and chicken.

You can use the crusts on individual 6- to 10-ounce fillets or larger 2½- to 4-pound fillets (that can serve ten to twelve), although cooking time will vary. You can pat crusts (of bread crumbs, nuts, vegetables, olives, or mixtures of these) onto a coating of mustard, vinaigrette, or even reduced-calorie maple syrup or a mayonnaise mixture. They provide low-calorie, hassle-free, heart-healthy alternatives to fish fries and fat-laden recipes.

Mustard Horseradish-Crusted
Arctic Char or Halibut

YIELD: 4 SERVINGS

Ingredients

4 boned fillets of Arctic char or halibut
  (½ pound per person)

¾ cup Dijon mustard

¾ cup white horseradish

¾ cup seasoned breadcrumbs

Fresh minced chives or parsley

1. Preheat oven to 350°F.
2. Place fillets skin side down on oiled pan.
3. Combine mustard and horseradish and rub on top of fillets.
4. Pat thickly with seasoned bread crumbs.
5. Bake 15 minutes.
6. Remove from oven and garnish with minced chives or finely chopped parsley.

Note: This recipe can be adapted to cod, sea trout, bass, and other whitefish fillets.

Panko-Crusted Sea Bass
with Tomato Provençal Sauce

YIELD: 4 SERVINGS

Tomato Provençal Sauce Ingredients

2 shallots, finely minced

6 cloves garlic, finely minced

1 teaspoon fresh cracked
  black pepper

¼ teaspoon crushed red pepper

¾ cup extra-virgin olive oil

1 teaspoon anchovy paste

¼ cup sherry vinegar

2 8-ounce cans tomatoes, diced

Salt to taste

Ground white pepper to taste

2 teaspoons snipped chives

2 teaspoons tarragon, minced

2 teaspoons chervil, minced

2 teaspoons parsley, minced

2 teaspoons basil, minced

1. In a sauté pan, sweat the shallots, garlic, cracked black pepper, and crushed red pepper in 2 tablespoons olive oil until the shallots are opaque in appearance.

2. Add the remaining olive oil, anchovy paste, sherry vinegar, and diced tomatoes. Whisk this mixture well and let simmer for 20 minutes.

3. Season with salt, white pepper, and all the herbs. Keep the sauce hot until needed.

Sea Bass Ingredients

2 pounds cleaned sea bass fillets

Salt to taste

Ground white pepper to taste

2 cups flour

3 eggs

2 ounces milk

2 cups panko breadcrumbs
  (or regular breadcrumbs)

2 cups pure olive oil

1. Cut sea bass into 4 equal portions of about 8 ounces each. Season with salt and ground white pepper.

2. Using a standard breading procedure, bread fish by dredging in flour first, then egg and milk wash, and then the breadcrumbs. (Once completed, you can keep the fish in the refrigerator for up to 2 hours.)

3. Preheat oven to 375°F. Heat pure olive oil in large sauté pan. Shallow-fry sea bass until golden brown.

4. Once golden brown, remove sea bass from oil, place on sheet pan, and finish in oven for five minutes or until fully cooked.

5. While the sea bass is in the oven, make sure the sauce is hot—then pour it over cooked sea bass.

Olive-Coated Bass with Tomato Herb Vinaigrette

YIELD: 4 SERVINGS

Tomato Herb Vinaigrette Ingredients

4 tomatoes

2 cloves garlic

1 teaspoon fresh thyme

2 tablespoons fresh basil

½ cup extra-virgin olive oil

Pinch black pepper

1–2 teaspoons sugar (or Splenda)

4 tablespoons red wine or sherry vinegar

2 teaspoons salt

Blend all in blender; use with grilled fish or on vegetables.

YIELD: 6 SERVINGS

Olive-Coated Bass Ingredients

6 fillets wild, sea, or farm-raised bass with skin (6–7 ounces each, about ¾ inch thick)

½ cup extra-virgin olive oil

4–6 anchovy fillets

2 tablespoons capers

1 tablespoon garlic, finely chopped (to taste)

1 teaspoon fresh minced thyme

2 teaspoons fresh minced parsley

1 tablespoon brandy

½–¾ cup breadcrumbs

½ cup parmesan cheese (preferably freshly grated)

Lemon zest from 1 lemon

1 cup pitted Kalamata, oil-cured, or other good-quality black olives, coarsely chopped

1. Preheat oven to 400°F.
2. Coat skin of bass with 1 to 2 tablespoons olive oil and sauté in hot pan, skin side down, for a few minutes until skin is well seared. Remove from pan and place skin side down in a shallow baking pan.
3. In a food processor, puree remainder of olive oil with anchovies, garlic, thyme, parsley, and brandy.
4. Spoon olive oil mixture on fish fillets.
5. Combine breadcrumbs, parmesan cheese, lemon zest, and olives.
6. Pat breadcrumb mixture onto fish fillets.
7. Bake 7 to 10 minutes (or just until fish flakes).
8. Serve with 2 to 3 tablespoons Tomato Herb Vinaigrette (see above).

Wildflower Crab Cake with Vanilla-Mango Chutney and Lemon Thyme Vinaigrette

Vanilla-Mango Chutney Ingredients

3 mangoes, diced very small

1 vanilla bean (extract seeds)

2 shallots, diced very small

1 tablespoon chopped chives

1 tablespoon white wine vinegar

In a mixing bowl, mix the mangoes with the vanilla bean, shallots, chives, and vinegar.

Lemon Thyme Vinaigrette Ingredients

Juice of 2 lemons

½ cup white wine vinegar

1 teaspoon chopped thyme

vegetable oil

In a bowl, mix lemon juice with chopped thyme and slowly add the oil until it emulsifies.

Wildflower Crab Cake Ingredients

16-ounce can fresh jumbo lump crabmeat

Zest of ½ lemon

Juice of ½ lemon

1 tablespoon mayonnaise

Salt and pepper

½ cup breadcrumbs

olive oil cooking spray

1. Preheat oven to 350°F.
2. Mix crabmeat with lemon zest, juice, mayonnaise, salt, pepper, and breadcrumbs. Do not overmix the crabmeat; otherwise, it will break up.
3. Mold into round cake shapes and dust with a little breadcrumbs.
4. Sear the cakes in a nonstick skillet sprayed with olive oil or vegetable spray until golden brown on each side.
5. Place in oven for 4 minutes until hot in the middle.
6. Serve over Vanilla-Mango Chutney, sprinkled with Lemon Thyme Vinaigrette.

Pan-Seared John Dory with Melted Leeks and Vanilla Sauce

John Dory fillet is a very exceptional fish that's not too hard to find. Ask a good fishmonger to locate some for you. It has a very delicate flavor and is very easy to cook.

YIELD: 4 SERVINGS

Ingredients

2 large leeks, washed (peel off the outer leaves)

¼ cup butter

2 shallots, peeled and sliced very thin

¼ cup blended oil

1 cup white wine

1 sprig thyme

1 dry bay leaf

5 black peppercorns

½ cup heavy whipping cream

1 fresh vanilla bean

4 John Dory fillets

Salt and pepper to taste

1. Cut leeks in half; then cut into very thin slices. Wash very well.
2. In a small sauté pan, melt butter on low heat and add leeks. Cook leeks very slowly until moist and tender, but do not lose the lovely greenness.
3. In another small pan, cook shallots in a small amount of oil.
4. Slowly cook; add white wine, thyme, bay leaf, and peppercorns.
5. When almost reduced, add cream, bring to a boil, and remove from heat.
6. Cut the vanilla bean in half lengthwise; scrape out the seeds inside, and add to cream. Let steep for about 5 minutes.
7. Strain the sauce very well, using a fine strainer. Reserve for later.
8. Heat a nonstick sauté pan. Season the fish with salt and pepper and add fish to the pan with a little oil.
9. Keep turning fish until golden brown; normally, it doesn't take long. Cook about 5 minutes.
10. Place melted leeks on the middle of the plate.
11. Place the John Dory on top of the leeks, and spoon the sauce around the plate.

Mussels Fra Diavolo

YIELD: 4 SERVINGS

Ingredients

2 tablespoons minced garlic

2 tablespoons olive oil

1 cup red wine

8 cups plum tomatoes, hand-crushed

2 cups chicken broth (optional)

½ teaspoon dried oregano

½ teaspoon dried basil

½ teaspoon crushed red pepper

4 dozen mussels

2 bay leaves

2 tablespoons fresh chopped parsley

1. Sauté garlic in olive oil.
2. Add red wine, plum tomatoes, chicken broth, dried herbs, and red pepper. Mix well.
3. Add mussels and simmer until they open (stir gently).
4. Add parsley right before serving.

Pistachio-Crusted Salmon

YIELD: 4 SERVINGS

Ingredients

4 salmon fillets (½ pound per person)

Salt and pepper to taste

½ cup reduced-calorie maple syrup

¾ cup chopped pistachio nuts

1. Preheat oven to 350°F.
2. Place fillets skin side down on oiled pan.
3. Sprinkle with salt and pepper to taste.
4. Rub maple syrup on top of fillets.
5. Dust with pistachio nuts.
6. Bake 10 to 15 minutes (to desired degree of doneness).

Scallion-Potato-Crusted Salmon

YIELD: 4 SERVINGS

Ingredients

2 tablespoons olive oil

2 bunches scallions (white and green parts), cut in ½-inch slices

2 cups mashed potatoes, seasoned with salt and white pepper

4 salmon fillets (½ pound per person)

Salt and pepper

1. Preheat oven to 350°F.
2. Heat oil in skillet and sauté scallions until wilted.
3. Mix scallions into mashed potatoes.
4. Place fillets skin side down on oiled pan.
5. Sprinkle with salt and pepper to taste.
6. Spread ½ cup mashed potatoes on each fillet.
7. Bake 15 minutes (to desired degree of doneness).

Hibachi Salmon with Soy and Sesame Glaze

YIELD: 4 SERVINGS

Ingredients

1 cup soy sauce

1 cup teriyaki sauce

½ cup orange juice

1 tablespoon garlic

1 tablespoon fresh ginger, minced

1 tablespoon cornstarch dissolved in ½ teaspoon water

4 salmon fillets (8 ounces each)

1 scallion, sliced

Black and white sesame seeds

1. In a saucepan, combine soy sauce, teriyaki sauce, orange juice, garlic, and ginger.
2. Bring to a boil; thicken with cornstarch and water mixture.
3. Spoon glaze over salmon and cook through. Salmon can be grilled, broiled, poached, or baked.
4. Garnish with sliced scallions and black and white sesame seeds.

Seared Scallops with Pomegranate Vinaigrette

Scallop Ingredients

12 each U10 diver scallops or U10 dry pack scallops

Kosher salt to taste

Ground white pepper to taste

2 ounces clarified butter or pure olive oil

1. Remove muscle tabs from scallops and place in small pot for sauce. Reserve scallops and bring to room temperature for cooking.
2. Heat a large sauté pan over high heat.
3. Season scallops with salt and ground white pepper.
4. Add clarified butter or oil to pan and place scallops in pan. Do not move scallops! Let cook about 1 to 2 minutes, or just until golden brown.
5. Turn over once and let cook until golden brown again.
6. Place on plate and drizzle with vinaigrette.

Pomegranate Vinaigrette Ingredients

1 cup pomegranate juice

1 cup honey

4 ounces grapeseed oil

Kosher salt to taste

Ground white pepper to taste

1. In a small saucepan, reduce pomegranate juice by three-quarters or until it has a light syrupy consistency. Remove from pot and place in small mixing bowl.
2. Add honey and combine well.
3. In a slow, steady stream, whisk in grapeseed oil to form an emulsion.
4. Season with salt and ground white pepper.
5. Reserve for plating. The vinaigrette can be made up to 3 days in advance and kept refrigerated.

Salmon Cakes, Many Ways

YIELD: 4 SERVINGS

Ingredients

16-ounce can salmon (preferably water-packed and red sockeye), drained well, with bones and skin removed, or 2 7-ounce cans or pouches of "skinless and boneless" salmon, or 1½ cups leftover cooked salmon

½ cup finely minced onion

2 tablespoons fresh lemon juice

2 egg whites, lightly beaten

¼ teaspoon salt

¼ teaspoon freshly ground pepper

Pinch cayenne pepper

1 cup saltine cracker crumbs or bread crumbs (see note below)

1 tablespoon olive oil

Lemon wedges

Chopped parsley

1. Flake salmon with a fork in mixing bowl.
2. Add onion, lemon juice, egg whites, salt, and peppers and mix lightly. Add just enough cracker crumbs to bind mixture (¼–½ cup).
3. Shape into 4 burgers and coat with remaining crumbs.
4. Place on cookie sheet that has been sprayed 2 to 3 times with olive or vegetable oil spray and refrigerate for 30 minutes or freeze for 10 minutes.
5. After brushing the top surface with olive oil, bake in a 375°F oven for 30 to 40 minutes until well browned or fry 4 to 5 minutes on each side in a hot nonstick skillet that has been sprayed with vegetable oil spray.
6. Serve with lemon wedges and chopped fresh parsley for garnish.

Note: You can make cracker crumbs or breadcrumbs in a food processor. Salmon cakes can be wrapped individually and frozen.

Variations

1. Instead of the minced onion, sauté 1 coarsely chopped Spanish onion and 1 large red pepper, diced, 5 to 6 minutes in 2 teaspoons olive oil in a nonstick skillet. Cool and add to cooked salmon mixture.
2. Add 1 package frozen chopped spinach (thawed, well drained) to the salmon mixture.
3. For the onion, you can substitute 1 bunch of scallions, including green tops, sliced into ¼-inch rounds and sautéed 2 to 3 minutes.

POULTRY

Coq au Vin–Style Chicken
Steve Topple

Roasted Meyer Lemon Chicken
Paul Ferzacca

The World's Best Grilled Chicken Burgers
Brian Peck

The Sage's Turkey Meatloaf Extraordinaire
(adapted from the Sage Restaurant)
Harriette Mogul

Traditional Turkey Meatloaf (adapted from James Coco)
Harriette Mogul

Tailgate Turkey Chili
Harriette Mogul

Stuffed Eggplant with Meat and Mushrooms
Harriette Mogul

Mushroom-Stuffed Chicken Breasts
Mark Kramer

Rosemary Tuscan Turkey Breast
Harriette Mogul

Chicken and turkey are low in fat and low in calories. But be sure to use only skinned chicken breasts for these recipes—and remove the fringe of fat that sometimes gets left behind in the packaging.

Ground turkey and chicken can have a higher fat content than you may imagine, so buy the products labeled "lean" or "all white meat."

Many supermarkets today have butcher counters where, for just a few pennies more per pound, you can get fresh-ground turkey or chicken and specify "lean" or ground breast only. This not only decreases the calories per pound but improves the taste of the meatballs and meatloaves that add variety to your diet.

I have a whole shelf of cookbooks devoted to chicken alone, and all of our Vail and Chappaqua chefs have many chicken breast recipes in their repertoires. Thus, I've included several of the most popular entrées—the ones lowest in calories and especially healthy.

Meatballs and meatloaves embody many of the concepts of this book. They are easy to prepare in large quantity and can be stored in individual or family-size servings as a basis for several future meals with minimal fuss and cleanup. Like braised meats and stews and other "slow foods" that yield an abundance of sauce, these dishes' flavors even improve when reheated the second time around, so they are perfect for busy women. Variants of meatballs are found in all cuisines of the world, and they are always big favorites of children and adults of all ages.

Here are several favorite meatball and meatloaf recipes, along with a few for chicken and turkey burgers. (I still cook these on those Sunday mornings when I want to stock my freezer or have a simple Sunday supper after a day of other activities.)

Coq au Vin–Style Chicken

This is a nice homey dish to make when it is cold outside; they sell lots of it in the restaurant.

YIELD: 4 SERVINGS

Ingredients

4 boneless, skinless chicken breasts

4 chicken legs

1 cup green onion, sliced in small strips

4 cloves garlic, peeled and crushed

6 dark plums, each cut into 8 pieces

2 cups pitted olives, cut in half

1 bottle chardonnay

2 cups white wine vinegar

Salt and pepper to taste

1. In a large ovenproof pot, sauté the chicken legs; add the green onion, garlic, plums, and olives.
2. Sauté for 10 minutes until golden brown.
3. Deglaze the pan with all the white wine and vinegar.
4. Reduce the wine by half and then add the chicken breast.
5. Season with salt and pepper.
6. If you need to add more liquid, just add a little water.
7. Put oiled parchment paper or foil on top and place in a warm oven at 350°F.
8. Cook for 45 minutes.
9. Remove from heat and serve 1 breast and 1 piece of leg per person.
10. Serve some of the juice on top.
11. If you want potatoes, sauté a couple of fingerling potatoes and serve.

Roasted Meyer Lemon Chicken

YIELD: 4 SERVINGS

Ingredients

1 farm-raised whole chicken
3 Meyer lemons
8 garlic cloves
2 4-inch sprigs fresh rosemary
4 sprigs fresh oregano
4 sprigs fresh Italian parsley

1 bay leaf
6 ounces extra-virgin olive oil
Kosher salt to taste
Ground black pepper to taste
1 tablespoon red wine vinegar

1. Preheat oven to 375°F.
2. Rinse chicken and pat dry.
3. Zest lemons with a vegetable peeler, and put zest inside of chicken cavity.
4. Cut lemons in half and juice into a small stainless-steel or glass bowl, and reserve juice for sauce.
5. Peel all garlic, place 5 cloves inside cavity of chicken, and mince 3 cloves; add the 3 minced cloves to lemon juice for sauce.
6. Place 1 4-inch sprig of rosemary inside cavity of chicken with garlic and lemon zest. Pick leaves from the other 4-inch sprig of rosemary and chop fine. Place in bowl with lemon juice.
7. Place 2 sprigs of oregano inside cavity of chicken. Pick leaves from the other 2 sprigs of oregano and chop fine. Place in bowl with lemon juice.
8. Place 2 sprigs of Italian parsley inside cavity of chicken. Chop the remaining 2 sprigs of Italian parsley and add to lemon juice.
9. Place bay leaf inside cavity of chicken.
10. Rub chicken with 2 ounces olive oil, and season chicken well inside and out with salt and ground black pepper.
11. Truss chicken with butcher's twine.
12. Place on roasting rack, breast side up, in a roasting pan.
13. Roast at 375°F until the thigh meat registers an internal temperature of 150°F, approximately 1 hour.
14. While chicken is roasting, finish lemon sauce:
15. Add to lemon juice and herbs 1 tablespoon red wine vinegar, kosher salt, and ground black pepper to taste, and whisk in remaining 4 ounces of olive oil. Check seasoning and adjust if necessary.

16. When the chicken thigh reaches an internal temperature of 150°F, remove chicken and let rest.
17. Clarify fat in the roasting pan, and discard all but 1 ounce of chicken fat.
18. Deglaze the pan with the lemon mixture.
19. Cut chicken into quarters and place back in roasting pan with lemon sauce; let cook another 5 minutes.
20. Serve on large platter and enjoy.

The World's Best Grilled Chicken Burgers

YIELD: 4 SERVINGS

Ingredients

2½ pounds chicken breasts
2 ounces Dijon mustard
1 ounce shallots, chopped fine

1 ounce fresh parsley, minced
1 ounce vegetable oil
Salt and pepper to taste

1. Place chicken in a food processor and process until smooth.
2. Add mustard, shallots, parsley, oil, salt, and pepper.
3. Make 4 patties.
4. Brush with vegetable oil.
5. Place on a preheated grill and cook until done, approximately 2 to 3 minutes per side.

The Sage's Turkey Meatloaf Extraordinaire

This recipe comes from the Sage Restaurant at the Aspen Sports Center. The Sage has a heart-healthy menu to accompany its spa. The meatloaf is low in calories and low in fat; I have made a few modifications.

YIELD: 16 SERVINGS

Ingredients

1½ cups chopped onions

1 cup chopped carrots

2 tablespoons finely minced garlic

2 tablespoons finely minced ginger

1–2 tablespoons flavored olive oil

1 cup minced red pepper

2 cups sliced mushrooms

¾ cup dried cranberries (or sun-dried tomatoes, cut up)

1⅓ cups breadcrumbs (preferably homemade or "Japanese" as in the original recipe)

1 cup Egg Beaters or 4 egg whites, slightly frothed

2 tablespoons sesame oil

½ cup soy sauce

Salt and pepper to taste

3½–5 pounds ground turkey

1–2 packages chopped spinach, thawed and drained (optional)

1. Sauté onions, carrots, garlic, and ginger in olive oil for 10 minutes (or until softened but not browned).
2. Add red pepper, mushrooms, and dried cranberries (or sun-dried tomatoes) and cook for an additional 5–10 minutes. Cool.
3. In large bowl, moisten breadcrumbs with Egg Beaters (or egg whites), sesame oil, and soy sauce.
4. Season with salt and pepper to taste. Let stand until moisture is absorbed.
5. Add ground turkey and spinach.
6. Fold in cooled cooked vegetables. (Handle lightly.)
7. Place in 2 12-inch-long greased loaf pans. (You can use an oil spray to mist the pan.) Or divide mixture in half and form into 2 large or 4 small meatloaves, and place side by side with at least 2 inches between each loaf in a large baking pan (for a more browned and crustier version).
8. Bake at 325°F for 1 to 1¼ hours. Do not overcook.

Variations

This also makes great meatballs. Gently shape them into 1½- to 2-inch-diameter meatballs and bake or broil them on a rack on a shallow baking sheet. Or simmer them for about 1 hour in any good-quality jarred marinara or other tomato sauce in a covered 4-quart pot.

Traditional Turkey Meatloaf

YIELD: 8 SERVINGS

Ingredients

1 cup fresh or packaged breadcrumbs
½ cup light sour cream
2 egg whites, lightly beaten
2 large garlic cloves, finely minced
2 teaspoons Worcestershire sauce (or other bottled steak sauce)
¼ cup chopped fresh dill (or 2 tablespoons dried dill weed)

½ teaspoon salt (preferably sea salt), or to taste
¼ teaspoon fresh ground pepper, or to taste
1 large onion, minced
1 cup mushrooms, chopped
1½ cups shredded carrots
2 pounds ground lean turkey (or veal)

1. Preheat oven to 350°F.
2. Place breadcrumbs, sour cream, egg whites, garlic, Worcestershire sauce, dill, salt, and pepper in large mixing bowl. Mix well and let stand for 5 to 10 minutes until crumbs absorb the liquid. Add onion, mushrooms, and carrots and combine.
3. Add ground meat, handling lightly. Mix just until combined.
4. Place into 1 large or 2 medium loaf pans.
5. Bake for 1¼ hours until top of meatloaf is firm to the touch and juices are clear.
6. Remove from oven and let stand at room temperature for 5 to 10 minutes before serving. Pour off liquid and reserve.
7. Invert onto warm platter, slice into ½-inch slices, and serve with reserved liquid.

Note: The meatloaf freezes well in the reserved juices. You can also eat it at room temperature.

Tailgate Turkey Chili

YIELD: 8 SERVINGS

Ingredients

1 pound lean ground turkey
3 tablespoons chili powder
2 teaspoons cumin powder
2 teaspoons dried oregano or thyme
Salt to taste
1 tablespoon olive oil
3 garlic cloves, peeled and chopped
   finely
1 large Spanish onion, coarsely
   chopped (reserve 2–4 tablespoons
   for garnish if desired)
1 large red pepper, cut in ½-inch
   pieces
4-ounce can mild green chilies or 2–4
   tablespoons finely minced fresh

jalapeño peppers (prepared from a
   large seeded jalapeño pepper that
   you mince wearing rubber gloves)
1 teaspoon crushed red pepper (or
   more to taste)
Freshly ground black pepper to taste
2 28-ounce cans quality whole or
   crushed tomatoes
15-ounce can kidney beans or black
   beans, drained and rinsed
Optional garnishes: 2 ounces shredded
   cheddar or other cheese, chopped
   fresh onion, fresh chopped parsley,
   or coriander

1. Cook turkey over medium heat in large sauté pan or saucepan, stirring frequently to crumble just until pink color is lost (5 to 6 minutes).
2. Place meat in a mesh strainer. Pour 1 to 2 cups of boiling water over meat to remove all fat. Set meat aside in a large mixing bowl.
3. Season meat with chili powder, cumin, oregano, and salt.
4. Pour off any fat from pan, and wipe with a paper towel.
5. Add olive oil to pan and heat 1 minute over medium heat.
6. Add minced garlic and cook for an additional minute.
7. Add onion and cook for an additional 5 minutes until onion becomes soft and translucent. Then add red pepper and cook for an additional 3 minutes.
8. Return meat to pan, add all additional ingredients, mix well, and correct seasonings.
9. Cook uncovered for 30 more minutes on top of the stove over low heat. Or you can transfer the mixture to an ovenproof saucepot or casserole with lid and cook in the oven at 350°F for 45 minutes. (Stir once during cooking.)

10. Serve over ½ cup boiled rice or a small baked potato.
11. Top each serving with chopped fresh onion or 1 to 2 tablespoons shredded cheddar or other cheese. Garnish with chopped fresh parsley or coriander as desired.

Note: You can easily double this recipe; it freezes well.

Stuffed Eggplant with Meat and Mushrooms

YIELD: 4 SERVINGS

Ingredients

2 medium eggplants
1 pound lean ground turkey or veal
1 tablespoon olive oil
2 large garlic cloves, finely minced
1 large Spanish onion, chopped
8 ounces fresh mushrooms, sliced
1 red bell pepper, cut into ½-inch pieces
1 teaspoon salt

Freshly ground pepper to taste
½ cup fresh or packaged seasoned breadcrumbs
2 beaten egg whites
1 cup canned tomatoes, chopped
½ cup grated parmesan cheese (optional)
¼ cup chopped fresh basil, chervil, or parsley

1. Preheat oven to 375°F.
2. Wash eggplants; cut in half lengthwise and remove pulp, leaving a ½-inch rim. (A melon ball scooper works well.) Reserve eggplant shells.
3. Sauté meat just until lightly browned in large nonstick frying pan. (Do not overcook.)
4. Remove meat from pan using a slotted spoon, and wipe excess fat from pan. Put meat aside in a bowl.
5. Heat olive oil over medium heat. Add garlic and cook for 2 minutes. Then add onion, mushrooms, eggplant, and red pepper and cook 6 to 8 minutes until softened.
6. Combine with meat in bowl. Season with salt and pepper.
7. Add breadcrumbs, egg whites, and tomatoes, and mix lightly. Spoon into eggplant shells.
8. Sprinkle with parmesan cheese (if desired).
9. Bake 35 to 45 minutes.
10. Sprinkle with fresh chopped basil, chervil, or parsley prior to serving.

Mushroom-Stuffed Chicken Breasts

YIELD: 6 SERVINGS

Ingredients

6 boneless, skinless chicken breasts

Salt and pepper to taste

3 cloves, plus one tablespoon, garlic, minced

¼ cup minced shallots

3 tablespoons extra-virgin olive oil

1 pound white button mushrooms, cleaned and coarsely chopped

1 cup white wine

1 teaspoon kosher salt

½ teaspoon freshly ground pepper

½ cup flour

2 eggs

½ cup Dijon mustard

2 cups breadcrumbs

¼ cup fresh parsley, finely chopped

1. Cut a slit, forming a pocket, from one end to the other of each chicken breast.
2. Season inside and out with salt, pepper, and 3 cloves minced garlic.
3. Sauté minced shallots in olive oil for a minute or so and add mushrooms.
4. Cook until mushrooms are soft and most liquid has evaporated.
5. Add 1 tablespoon minced garlic, wine, salt, and pepper; continue to cook until all moisture evaporates. Cool.
6. Fill each chicken breast with the mushroom filling.
7. Dredge each stuffed breast carefully in flour, then in combined egg and mustard mixture, and lightly coat with combined breadcrumbs and parsley.
8. Place on a lightly greased baking sheet; bake at 375°F for 20 minutes or until chicken is thoroughly cooked.

Rosemary Tuscan Turkey Breast

Ingredients

4–6 large sprigs fresh rosemary, washed and patted dry

4–6 cloves garlic, peeled and sliced in ¼-inch slices

1 3- to 4-pound boned and tied turkey breast with skin (have butcher prepare it)

Sea salt and freshly ground pepper to taste

2 large Spanish onions, peeled and sliced into ½-inch slices

2 large Yukon Gold potatoes, peeled and sliced into ½-inch slices

1. One day prior to cooking, insert rosemary sprigs and garlic slices in the pockets and under the skin of the turkey breast, created by gently loosening the skin.
2. Rub sea salt and freshly ground pepper on the skin and over all the exposed areas of the turkey breast. Cover with plastic wrap and refrigerate overnight or for 1 to 2 days.
3. Preheat oven to 375°F.
4. Prepare a large Reynolds oven bag according to directions for conventional oven on the package.
5. Place a layer of onion slices on the bottom of the cooking bag.
6. Next, layer the potato slices.
7. Finally, place the turkey breast, skin side up, on top of the vegetables.
8. Tie bag and place in a flat 9 × 13-inch pan, according to directions on the cooking bag.
9. Roast for 2 hours until turkey skin is golden brown or until an instant-read thermometer reaches an internal temperature of 160°F. (You can plunge the thermometer right into the middle of the breast through the plastic bag after 1½ hours.) Do not overcook or the turkey will be dry.
10. Remove from oven and let sit undisturbed for 15 to 20 minutes.
11. Carefully slit top of bag open and remove turkey breast to wooden platter or cutting board. Using kitchen shears, cut away butcher's ties and remove rosemary sprigs and garlic (if desired). Remove and discard the turkey skin and carve turkey breast into ¼- to

(continued)

Rosemary Tuscan Turkey Breast (*continued*)

½-inch slices, and serve with onions, potato slices, and gravy.
(You may puree the onions with the pan juices in a food processor
if you prefer a thicker gravy.)

12. Before freezing, place remaining gravy in refrigerator or freezer
to allow you to separate the fat that may form on the top from the
remainder of the gravy.

13. Store leftover turkey and onions in remaining gravy.

Variations

1. Brining: Instead of a dry rub before cooking, you can brine
the turkey for 1 to 2 days in a mixture of salt, water, garlic, and
rosemary. Dry well before cooking.

2. Vegetable substitute: Instead of potatoes, you can substitute carrots
halved lengthwise and cut into 2-inch lengths.

3. Bone-in turkey breast: You may substitute a single or double bone-
in turkey breast, which will require additional cooking time. To
avoid overcooking the vegetables, use peeled individual fingerling
potatoes. Slice the onions 1-inch thick, and don't cut the carrots in
half lengthwise before cutting into 2-inch lengths.

SIDE DISHES AND VEGETABLES

Asparagus with Truffle Butter and Fleur de Sel
Mark Kramer

Beautiful Broccoli and Pea Puree
Harriette Mogul

Roasted Carrots and Shallots
Mark Kramer

Haricots Verts Provençal
Paul Ferzacca

Wild Mushroom Sauté
Paul Ferzacca

Low-Fat Creamed Spinach
Mark Kramer

Julienned Vegetables with Shallot Butter Sauce
Brian Peck

Slow-Roasted Tomatoes
Paul Ferzacca

Asparagus with Truffle Butter and Fleur de Sel

YIELD: 4 SERVINGS

Ingredients

4 quarts water

1 tablespoon kosher salt

2 bunches thin fresh asparagus
   (bottom third removed)

1 tablespoon butter, melted

2 teaspoons black truffle paste
   (found in gourmet shops)

½ teaspoon fleur de sel (or other
   French sea salt)

¼ teaspoon freshly ground black pepper

1. Bring water and kosher salt to a boil.
2. Add asparagus and cook until barely tender, about 3 minutes. Drain.
3. Combine butter and truffle paste.
4. Transfer to platter and drizzle with butter/truffle paste mixture.
5. Sprinkle with fleur de sel, and finish with freshly ground black pepper. Toss lightly.

Beautiful Broccoli and Pea Puree

YIELD: 8 SERVINGS

Ingredients

2 large bunches broccoli

2 tablespoons butter (preferably unsalted)

2 tablespoons light cream or half-and-half

2 teaspoons salt (or more to taste)

1 teaspoon freshly ground black or white pepper (to taste)

2 packages frozen baby peas

1. Remove bottom inch of broccoli stalks and broccoli florets (leaving a ½-inch stem on each floret). Using a sharp knife or a vegetable peeler, remove tough fibrous outer edge of the broccoli stalks; slice crosswise into ½-inch slices.
2. Place broccoli stalks in a food steamer. Steam for 5 to 10 minutes until soft.
3. Remove broccoli from stove and place in bowl of food processor.
4. Steam broccoli florets for 4 to 5 minutes until soft.
5. Set aside half of the florets to be used as a topping for the puree. (You can cover these florets with 1 to 2 dozen ice cubes to maintain green color. Drain well after they cool and set aside. Reheat in steamer just prior to use.)
6. Add remaining half of the broccoli florets to the bowl of the food processor. Pulse to chop broccoli mixture; then add butter, cream, salt, and pepper, and puree until smooth.
7. Remove mixture from food processor bowl to a large mixing bowl. (Do not wash the food processor bowl.)
8. Defrost and heat peas in microwave or on top of the stove, according to package directions.
9. Drain peas and immediately puree in the food processor.
10. Using a rubber scraper, remove contents, add to broccoli mixture, and combine well. Add additional salt and pepper to taste.
11. Reheat puree in top of double boiler. Place in an oval or round gratin dish. (You can also reheat the puree in a 2- or 3-quart soufflé or gratin dish covered with aluminum foil in a 350°F oven for 20 to 30 minutes. Remove carefully from oven prior to next step.)

(continued)

Beautiful Broccoli and Pea Puree (*continued*)

12. Place broccoli florets that have been reheated in steamer (or microwave oven) on top of pureed broccoli (prettiest when arranged in an outer ring with the puree showing in the middle).

Note: This makes a beautiful presentation for holiday meals. For faster preparation, just combine all the broccoli and the peas (skip steps 5 and 12, and in step 6, add all the florets to the food processor). Either puree can be made in advance and freezes well.

Roasted Carrots and Shallots

YIELD: 4 SERVINGS

Ingredients

2 pounds fresh carrots, peeled and cut into ¼-inch slices

12 shallots, peeled and sliced

1 tablespoon chopped fresh parsley

1 teaspoon minced garlic

1 teaspoon kosher salt

¼ teaspoon freshly ground pepper

2 tablespoons extra-virgin olive oil

1. Preheat oven to 400°F.
2. Toss all ingredients together and place on a baking sheet.
3. Roast in oven until carrots are nicely caramelized and soft, about 20 to 30 minutes. Stir frequently so that they brown evenly.

Haricots Verts Provençal
(French Green Beans Cooked with Tomatoes, Garlic, Basil, and Olive Oil)

Ingredients

4 Roma tomatoes

24 ounces haricots verts (French green beans)

3 shallots, minced

8 garlic cloves, minced

4 ounces extra-virgin olive oil

½ cup chopped fresh basil

Kosher salt to taste

Ground white pepper to taste

1. Fill a 2-gallon pot with water and bring to a boil.
2. Using a small paring knife, remove stem from each Roma tomato and score an X on the other end of tomato to prepare for blanching to remove skin and seeds.
3. Remove ends of the haricots verts, and reserve for blanching.
4. Set up an ice bath with plenty of ice and cold water to refresh the tomatoes and haricots verts once blanched.
5. Once the water is at a rolling boil, blanch the Roma tomatoes for about 15 seconds to just blister the skin, and refresh in the ice bath.
6. Remove from ice bath; let drain. Keep ice bath to refresh haricots verts.
7. Season the boiling water with enough salt to make it taste like the ocean. This will retain the color of the beans when cooking. *Note*: Green vegetables release acid into the water, and the evaporation will discolor the vegetables. To counteract the acid, add an alkali to the water (salt is an excellent alkali). Don't cover the pot, or the acid released in evaporation will be dispersed back into the water.
8. After the water is back at a rolling boil and seasoned with salt, blanch the haricots verts for about 5 minutes or until al dente. The starches should be jelled completely when cooking any bean, to aid in the digestion process.
9. Remove beans and refresh in the ice bath. Once chilled, again remove from water; let drain well. This step can be done 1 day in advance.

(continued)

Haricots Verts Provençal
(French Green Beans Cooked with Tomatoes, Garlic, Basil, and Olive Oil)
(*continued*)

10. Prepare the tomatoes: Remove skin, cut into quarters lengthwise, and remove seeds. Then dice the tomato quarters into ¼-inch pieces and reserve. You can do this a day in advance.
11. Clean and peel the shallots and garlic. Finely dice the shallots and mince the garlic, and reserve each separately. You can do this a day in advance.
12. To finish cooking the Haricots Verts Provençal, bring a large sauté pan to medium heat; add olive oil, shallots, garlic, and haricots verts. Let cook about 2 minutes, stirring frequently.
13. After 2 minutes, add the diced tomatoes and fresh basil; let cook another 2 minutes.
14. Season with kosher salt and ground white pepper to taste.

Wild Mushroom Sauté

These mushrooms are truly ambrosial and can be used as an appetizer, a side dish, or a topping for grilled fish, chicken, or meats.

Ingredients

2 tablespoons olive oil or 1 tablespoon olive oil and 1 tablespoon butter

2 shallots, minced

3–4 garlic cloves, minced

8 ounces wild mushrooms (mixture of shiitakes, oyster mushrooms, and chanterelles)

Sea salt to taste

Freshly ground white pepper to taste

Fines herbes (mixture of freshly chopped parsley, chervil, tarragon, and chives) or chopped parsley or minced chives

1. Heat oil in large skillet. Add shallots and garlic, and sauté for 2 to 3 minutes over high heat.
2. Add mushrooms in 4 separate mounds that you have flattened with a spatula. Make sure you leave space between them; do not crowd into a smaller pan.
3. Cook, without disturbing the mounds, over high heat for a minimum of 4 minutes, until the mushrooms have released their liquids and are well browned.
4. Using a flat spatula, carefully turn the mushroom mounds. Add salt and pepper and continue to cook until they are well browned on both sides.
5. Garnish with fines herbes and serve immediately.

Low-Fat Creamed Spinach

YIELD: 4 SERVINGS

Ingredients

1 cup 1 percent milk

½ teaspoon sea salt

¼ teaspoon freshly ground pepper

1 tablespoon cornstarch dissolved in
    ¼ cup 1 percent cold milk

1 clove garlic, minced

10-ounce package frozen chopped
    spinach (thawed, all water
    squeezed out)

½ cup fresh breadcrumbs mixed with
    1 tablespoon olive oil or melted
    butter (optional)

1. Heat milk to boiling with sea salt and pepper.
2. Whisk in combined cornstarch and milk mixture.
3. Boil 1 minute, whisking constantly.
4. Stir in garlic and spinach, and continue to cook on low heat until spinach is heated. Remove from heat and serve immediately.
5. If desired, you can put spinach in a gratin dish sprayed with vegetable oil spray, top mixture with crumbs, and place under the broiler for a few minutes until browned. Watch carefully.

Note: You can make this recipe with 2 packages of spinach for a lower-calorie version.

Julienned Vegetables
with Shallot Butter Sauce

YIELD: 4 SERVINGS

Ingredients

*Any combination of first four vegetables to
equal 3–4 cups, raw*
Carrots
Yellow squash
Zucchini

Broccoli florets
1 red onion
1 tablespoon butter
1 shallot, minced
Salt and pepper to taste

1. Julienne carrots, squash, and zucchini by hand (food processor will cut vegetables too small).
2. Slice red onion.
3. Cut broccoli into bite-size pieces.
4. Steam vegetables until tender, approximately 5 to 8 minutes.
5. Melt butter in large skillet and sauté shallot until translucent, about 2 minutes.
6. Add steamed vegetables to skillet and stir to mix.
7. Season with salt and pepper.

Slow-Roasted Tomatoes

YIELD: 8 SERVINGS

Ingredients

8 Roma tomatoes

8 yellow tomatoes

2 shallots, minced

6 garlic cloves, minced

1 tablespoon fresh thyme

Kosher salt to taste

Ground black pepper to taste

2 ounces extra-virgin olive oil

1. Preheat oven to 200°F.
2. Cut tomatoes in eighths. Place in large stainless-steel bowl.
3. Mince shallots and garlic; add to tomatoes.
4. Clean leaves from stems of fresh thyme; add leaves to tomatoes.
5. Season tomatoes with kosher salt and ground black pepper. Taste for quality.
6. Place tomatoes on a roasting rack on top of sheet pan, preferably, or directly on sheet pan. Drizzle with olive oil.
7. Cook in oven approximately 4 hours or until semidry.

NOT-SO-FORBIDDEN
FRUIT DESSERTS

Fuji Apple and Asian Pear Crisp with Blue Crumb Topping
Allana Smith

Baked Braeburn Apples with Sun-Dried Cider-Soaked Fruits
Allana Smith

Crispy Honey Nests with
Chèvre-Mascarpone Cream and Bing Cherries
Allana Smith

Concord Grape and Burgundy Poached Pears
with Quinoa Crisp Cookies
Allana Smith

Ricotta Ice Cream with Fresh Fruit in Lemon Verbena Syrup
Allana Smith

Raspberries au Gratin
Harriette Mogul

Cranberry-Raspberry Crisp
Jennifer and Harriette Mogul

Thanksgiving Treats
Harriette Mogul

Jenny's Cranberry-Raspeberry Conserve
Jennifer Mogul

Savor fresh, seasonal produce picked at its peak, accompanied by just a bit of pastry and a small portion of cream, custard, or cheese, and you'll find that these fruit-based desserts can satisfy the soul more fully than gooey, rich concoctions that grace most menus. The highlights—highly original combinations that are true first editions—represent the creative genius of Allana Smith, pastry chef at Larkspur.

As is the case with recipes in prior sections, you can repartition individual elements, like the Tazo tea and cider poaching syrup for the apples, the blue cheese topping for the pears, and the quinoa crisp cookies.

Just a bit of butter, cream, honey, or cheese characterizes each recipe, and you can decalorize all of them by halving the butter, substituting Splenda for sugar, or using reduced-calorie maple syrup in place of honey. But, unlike other recipes in the book, you'll probably discover that substitutions do compromise flavor. Remember the words of Dr. William Castelli, visionary researcher who first reported the association of dietary fat with heart disease in the legendary Framingham Report, and who noted in the *New York Times*, "Occasional tablespoons of real whipped cream or mayonnaise are preferable to ersatz versions."

Fuji Apple and Asian Pear Crisp
with Blue Crumb Topping

YIELD: 8 SERVINGS

Apple Pear Filling Ingredients

¼ cup butter

5 Fuji apples, peeled, cored, and sliced
⅛-inch thick

3 Asian pears, peeled, cored, and
sliced ⅛-inch thick

¼ cup granulated sugar

¼ cup honey

1 tablespoon flour

Juice of ½ lemon

¼ teaspoon cardamom

¼ teaspoon cloves

½ teaspoon cinnamon

1. Heat large, shallow sauté pan over medium-high heat.
2. Place butter in hot sauté pan; add apples, pears, and sugar, stirring occasionally. Cook until pears and apples soften slightly.
3. Add other ingredients to apples and pears and cook 1 more minute. Remove from heat and let fruits cool.
4. At this point, you can place the fruit mixture in a covered plastic container and store in the refrigerator up to 4 days, to be used whenever you need it.

Blue Crumb Topping Ingredients

1½ cups rolled oats

½ cup brown sugar

¾ cup Point Reyes Original blue cheese
(crumbled)

¼ cup cold butter, cubed

⅓ cup flour

1 teaspoon cinnamon

1 teaspoon salt

1. Combine all ingredients in the mixing bowl of an electric mixer; using the paddle attachment, mix until combined yet still crumbly.
2. At this point, you can put the topping in a covered plastic container and store in the refrigerator up to 4 days, to use as needed.

To Assemble and Bake

1. Preheat oven to 350°F.
2. Place fruit filling in the bottom three-fourths of either 8 6-ounce ramekins or 1 8-inch round or square cake pan.
3. Top with crumb topping.
4. Bake approximately 10 minutes. Serve hot, with (or without) a small scoop of vanilla bean ice cream.

Baked Braeburn Apples with Sun-Dried Cider-Soaked Fruits

YIELD: 8 SERVINGS

Fruit Topping Ingredients

½ cup dried cherries

½ cup dried cranberries

⅓ cup dates, halved and sliced thin

⅓ cup dried apricots, diced into
    very small pieces

⅓ cup dried figs, sliced

4 cups cider

2 tablespoons brown sugar

½ vanilla bean
    (scrape seeds into mixture)

2 tablespoons honey

1. Combine cherries, cranberries, dates, apricots, figs, 2 cups cider, brown sugar, vanilla bean seeds, and honey in small saucepan.
2. Bring to a boil, and boil for 20 minutes, or until rehydrated.
3. Strain out fruit and reserve.
4. Put other 2 cups cider in pan, and boil until reduced by half.
5. Add reduced sauce back to fruit mixture; cool.

Baked Apples Ingredients

8 Braeburn apples

3 Tazo Passion tea bags steeped
    in 4 cups cider (will work with
    plain water as well)

8 teaspoons butter

Brown sugar

1. Preheat oven to 350°F.
2. Cut apples in half vertically.
3. Use large end of a melon baller to scoop out core from both halves of each apple.
4. Make small slice on rounded side of each apple half so that it will sit flat later on.
5. Place cored-side down in a shallow baking dish and pour about 2–3 cups Passion cider over apples.
6. Bake in oven for 15 minutes (check pan after 10 minutes and add remaining cider as needed).
7. Flip each apple half and put ½ teaspoon butter in each half; sprinkle with brown sugar.
8. Bake 10 more minutes.
9. Let cool in pan; you can reheat apples in microwave or oven when you're ready to serve.
10. Serve 2 halves per person (one side up) with fruit topping.

Crispy Honey Nests with Chèvre-Mascarpone Cream and Bing Cherries

This is Allana's original recipe. A unique and spectacular dessert, this one is well worth the effort. All parts can be prepared in advance and assembled just prior to serving. We include options for decalorizing, but you may prefer to make the exact version for special occasions.

YIELD: 8 SERVINGS

Honey Nests Ingredients

8 metal rings, 2-inch diameter, 2 inches tall (you can make the nests without these, but the appearance will be flatter)

½ package (or ½ pound) kataifi (shredded filo dough)

½ cup melted butter

4 tablespoons sugar (or Splenda)

¼ cup wildflower honey

½ cup water

1. Preheat oven to 350°F.
2. Spread metal rings 2 inches apart on a parchment-lined baking sheet.
3. Pull a small handful of kataifi out of bag; wrap it around two of your fingers to form a "nest" that will fit into one of the rings. Repeat with every ring.
4. Using a pastry brush, brush approximately 1 tablespoon melted butter onto each kataifi "nest" and then sprinkle with ½ tablespoon sugar.
5. Place tray in oven; bake 10 to 15 minutes until golden brown.
6. Remove from oven. Let cool and remove rings.
7. Combine honey and water in a small saucepan on low heat until mixture boils; remove and cool.
8. Dip top of each nest in honey syrup. Set nests right side up on a clean, parchment-lined baking sheet.
9. When you finish the above step, pour any excess honey syrup onto the nests.
10. Return to oven for 5 minutes. Cool.

(continued)

Crispy Honey Nests with Chèvre-Mascarpone Cream and Bing Cherries (*continued*)

Chèvre-Mascarpone Cream Ingredients

17-ounce container mascarpone

4 ounces nonfat cream cheese

4 ounces quality chèvre

½ vanilla bean, seeds from scraping only

1 teaspoon finely grated orange zest

3 tablespoons lavender honey

1. Combine all ingredients with an electric mixer with the paddle attachment until just combined.
2. When you're ready to serve, scoop or pipe about ¼ cup of cheese mixture on top of each nest.
3. Top with preserved bing cherries or other preserved or fresh fruits.

Concord Grape and Burgundy Poached Pears with Quinoa Crisp Cookies

YIELD: 25 CRISPS

Poached Pears Ingredients

5 cups grape juice	1 cinnamon stick
3 cups red burgundy	Zest from ½ orange
1 vanilla bean	8 Bartlett pears, slightly hard

1. Combine grape juice, burgundy, and vanilla bean, cinnamon stick, and orange zest in 6- to 8-quart stockpot.
2. Peel pears and keep whole.
3. Place pears in pot with liquid and add more grape juice or water or wine until pears are completely submerged.
4. Top with a pot lid that is smaller in diameter than your pot. Put the lid directly on top of the pears to keep them submerged.
5. Depending on how soft the pears are, they take ½ hour to 1½ hours to cook at a slow simmer. To test doneness, poke a pear with a paring knife; it should insert very easily if pear is done.
6. Remove pears from heat, and remove with a slotted spoon into a baking pan to cool.
7. When cool, use a melon baller to scoop out the core of the pear from the bottom center of the stem.
8. You can keep pears up to one week in a covered container, refrigerated.
9. Return all of the poaching liquid to a saucepan, and heat on medium until it is reduced to thin syrup. Cool and store the sauce in an airtight container in refrigerator.

(continued)

Quinoa Crisps Ingredients

¾ cup quinoa

1½ cups rolled oats

½ cup sunflower seeds

½ cup raw pistachios, chopped fine

1 cup dried apricots, thinly sliced

½ cup honey

½ teaspoon salt

2 eggs

1½ teaspoons vanilla extract

2 tablespoons vegetable oil

1 egg white

1. Preheat oven to 350°F.
2. Rinse and strain quinoa; cook in 1½ cups boiling water.
3. Reduce to a simmer. Cook 12 minutes covered.
4. Spread quinoa on a baking sheet and bake until golden, stirring a few times.
5. Toast oats and sunflower seeds on a baking sheet in oven until lightly browned (about 5–10 minutes at 350°F); add to quinoa.
6. Reduce oven to 300°F.
7. Add nuts, apricots, ¼ cup honey, and salt to quinoa mix and cool.
8. Combine eggs, remaining ¼ cup honey, and vanilla, and add to quinoa mix.
9. Lightly spray parchment-lined baking sheet with vegetable spray.
10. Drop batter by rounded tablespoons onto parchment and spread to less than ¼-inch thick.
11. Bake 25 minutes at 300°F until crisp.
12. Cool and peel off of parchment. Store in an airtight container.

YIELD: 8 SERVINGS

Vanilla Bean Yogurt Sauce Ingredients

1 cup low-fat yogurt

2 tablespoons lavender honey

1 tablespoon vanilla extract

½ vanilla bean, scraped

Whisk ingredients together in a small bowl. To serve, spoon some of each sauce onto serving plates. Place 1 quinoa crisp on each plate and top with a whole poached pear. Drizzle pear with a little more of the reduced poaching liquid. Serve.

Ricotta Ice Cream with Fresh Fruit in Lemon Verbena Syrup

YIELD: ½ GALLON ICE CREAM, ENOUGH TO
SERVE 8 PEOPLE AND HAVE 2 PINTS LEFT OVER

Ricotta Ice Cream Ingredients

1½ cups sugar
1 cup water
3 cups high-quality ricotta
    cheese (I prefer Old Chatham

Shepherding Company's Sheep's
Milk Ricotta)
2 tablespoons honey
Pinch kosher salt

1. Stir sugar and water together in a small saucepan, and place on low heat.
2. Cook until all sugar is dissolved.
3. Set aside to cool.
4. Combine ricotta, honey, and salt in a food processor and process until smooth.
5. Place cheese mixture in a mixing bowl and whisk in the simple syrup. The ice cream is now ready to churn in an ice-cream machine (follow manufacturer's instructions).

Lemon Verbena Syrup Ingredients

2 cups water
2 cups sugar (or Splenda)
3 whole sprigs lemon verbena (or lemon zest, fresh mint, or lemon thyme)

1. Combine all ingredients in a small saucepan.
2. Over low heat, cook until sugar is dissolved.
3. Allow syrup to cool completely; then strain to remove lemon verbena.
4. Use just a few tablespoons of this syrup to flavor fresh fruit.
5. You can keep extra syrup refrigerated for 2 to 3 weeks.
6. Serve ice cream with fresh seasonal fruits tossed in Lemon Verbena Syrup (in winter, tropical fruits and citrus; in summer, berries, peaches, cherries, and plums).

Raspberries au Gratin

Ingredients

2 tablespoons unsalted softened butter, or almond, walnut, or hazelnut oil

4 pints fresh raspberries

½ teaspoon freshly grated nutmeg (optional)

2 cups heavy cream

½ cup dark brown sugar

1. Preheat broiler.
2. Rub softened butter or oil on 8 individual ramekins or a large oval gratin dish that can sustain high heat from a broiler.
3. Carefully layer ½ cup raspberries in each ramekin (or all in a single gratin dish).
4. Add nutmeg to cream and pour ¼ cup cream onto each ramekin.
5. Sprinkle each with 1 tablespoon brown sugar.
6. Broil 4 inches from heat for a few minutes, just until top is caramelized. Watch carefully.
7. Remove from broiler and let cool slightly before serving.

Cranberry-Raspberry Crisp

1. Double the recipe for Jenny's Cranberry-Raspberry Conserve, following the directions on page 242.
2. Make the oat topping by Allana Smith on page 233, omitting the blue cheese.
3. Preheat oven to 350°F.
4. Place cranberry mixture in 10- to 12-inch oval glass or porcelain gratin dish.
5. Top with crumb topping.
6. Bake for 10 minutes.
7. Serve warm with a small scoop or no-sugar-added vanilla ice cream or frozen yogurt or with Allana's ricotta ice cream on page 239.

Thanksgiving Treats

What to eat to be part of the party yet avert any aftermath:

- Only vegetables and seafood hors d'oeuvres (avoid all others)
- Lots of turkey without the skin (white meat is less caloric)
- One large spoonful of stuffing
- Mushrooms in the mushroom gravy (spare the sauce and skip any other gravies made from the drippings because they are always greasy and fat filled unless a fat separator has been used to skim off extra calories)
- As many green vegetables as possible (volunteer to bring string beans with almonds, broccoli with garlic crumbs, or roasted or steamed asparagus)
- Orange vegetables that aren't overly sweet, or a small spoonful of any others
- Small spoonful of cranberry sauce unless you use Jenny's Cranberry-Raspberry Conserve.
- Small piece apple or pumpkin pie without the crust with a rounded tablespoon of whipped cream (have only one dessert)
- Limit alcohol to a glass of dry white wine, red wine, or "lite" beer

Watch out for everything else, especially other alcoholic beverages, salted nuts, chips, dips, spreads, cheeses, candy, cookies, and cake!

Jenny's Cranberry-Raspberry Conserve

This is great with turkey at Thanksgiving—but also wonderful year-round served with yogurt, no-sugar-added ice cream, or in a crisp made with oat crumbs. Cranberries have five times the antioxidants of broccoli!

Ingredients

1 12-ounce bag fresh cranberries
½ cup water
1 cup Splenda Granulated
1 pint fresh raspberries

1. Combine cranberries, water, and Splenda in a medium saucepan.
2. Bring to a boil over medium heat, and simmer for 10 minutes, stirring occasionally.
3. Layer raspberries in an 8" × 8" Pyrex pan.
4. Carefully ladle warm cranberry mixture over raspberries.
5. Cool to room temperature.
6. Cover and refrigerate until ready to serve.

About the Chefs

Westchester Chefs

PHILIP CALLACI, executive chef and owner, and ANN CALLACI, founder, Penelope's Country Kitchen (Chappaqua, New York), and Dr. Produce (Armonk, New York)

The Callaci family moved to Chappaqua, New York, forty years ago, and just a few years later, Ann Callaci opened Dr. Produce in neighboring Armonk, the very first gourmet store in Upper Westchester to feature peak-of-the-market fruits and vegetables, "homemade" baked goods, and superhealthy takeout. Dr. Produce was my first call after inviting friends for dinner, so I got to know Ann over the years while picking up the grilled vegetables and wonderful dips that were part of my regular menu for summer entertaining.

Penelope's has expanded and now includes a soup/salad bar and an old-fashioned ice-cream stand. Fortunately, it continues in its original tradition, serving low-calorie, healthy, and imaginative salads, entrées, and side dishes.

JOE DI MAURO, owner, and JOHN EVERIN, chef, Mount Kisco Seafood and the Fish Cellar Restaurant (Mount Kisco, New York)

Joe Di Mauro grew up in Bedford, New York, with weekend forays behind his buddy's fish counter before he bought Mount Kisco Seafood (MKSF) in the late 1970s. In a single spectacular year, as he tells it, he acquired a house, a baby, and a store. Mount Kisco Seafood is the culmination of his intrigue with the sea, love of fish, and creative genius; it's a symbol of deceptive simplicity, reminiscent of summers at the shore and small-town USA.

Ten years ago, John Everin took over as executive chef, and thanks to Joe's vision, MKSF expanded to include a restaurant, the Fish Cellar, in downtown Mount Kisco, and a large catering division. Now, after thirty years, MKSF features a sushi chef, organic vegetables from nearby farms, and all the best accompaniments to the fantastic fresh fish from local waters and from the fish market in New York. Basically, we see no end in sight as Joe rewrites the American idiom from "a chicken in every pot" to "a fish on every plate."

SUSAN LAWRENCE (in memoriam) and Mark Kramer, executive chef, creative director, and proprietor, Susan Lawrence Catering (Chappaqua, New York)

Susan Lawrence started the tasty, tasteful takeout trend in Chappaqua more than two decades ago.

Recently honored as Best Caterer by *Westchester Magazine*, Mark Kramer has coordinated events for Bill and Hillary Clinton, the French Embassy in Washington, D.C., the *New York Times*, the Rockefeller family, Brooke Astor, Lady Bird Johnson, and a long list of celebrities. His extensive knowledge of food and keen sense of design drawn from the visual arts and cultural history are the culmination of a culinary career as a major Chicago pastry chef. The recipes he has graciously provided for this book are favorites from the shop that are both easy to prepare and superhealthy.

BRIAN PECK, executive chef, Satisfied Customer Catering Group, Katonah Grill (Katonah), McArthur's Grille, and Michael's Tavern (Pleasantville), Peabody's Café (Chappaqua and Valhalla Station, New York)

Brian Peck's food is the backbone of my diet, and McArthur's is my home away from home after long hours at the office. Brian cooked for President Bill Clinton and catered private parties for the U.S. Secret Service. Today, he has a wide following in the five restaurants where he oversees kitchens; diners love the homey taste of his food, his reliance on fresh ingredients, and his creative flair with comfort fare.

Brian's recipes are ideal for the carbohydrate-conscious home cook. Wonderfully homemade, they are the legacy of his mother's friends (first developed after Brian took over his family's cooking at age thirteen, following his mother's untimely death) and later refined at the CIA (the Culinary Institute of America) and in the kitchen of one of Zagat's highest-rated restaurants in Westchester.

I send a special thanks to Joanne, Brian's wife, who pushed Brian to pen them before she put them all on disc to share with *Syndrome W* readers.

GIONA STANCO and MARION MAZZELLA, chef and owner, Giona's Classic Tuscan Kitchen (Chappaqua, New York)

Giona's Classic Tuscan Kitchen opened in October 1996. Its owners—chef Giona Stanco and his mother, Marion Mazzella—learned and perfected the subtleties of Tuscan cuisine in Florence, Italy, where Giona was born and raised.

Giona's Classic Tuscan Kitchen is an eatery that specializes in simple food preparation, using the freshest market ingredients. Driven by their Florentine heritage, the owners strive to produce healthful, flavorful dishes "with few ancillary elements to detract from the integrity of the main ingredients."

Their beautiful store features fresh vegetables, along with a list of daily healthy "spa" and vegetarian soups, homemade pasta, and entrées and salads to transport patrons back to the banks of the Arno.

As they say in Giona's hometown of Firenze, *"Le donne sono deliziose, ma il cibo e' squisito!"* Women are delicious, but food is exquisite.

Vail Chefs

PAUL FERZACCA, proprietor and executive chef, La Tour

Paul Ferzacca came to Vail, Colorado, from Chicago, where, while working in kitchens at Spiaggia and the Ritz-Carlton, he was at the forefront of the culinary revolution that has overtaken that city in the past decade. Now owner and executive chef at La Tour, he oversees the restaurant voted "Best French Food in Vail" for several years running.

But this is not your father's French food. Paul's menu exemplifies how simple vegetables and widely available ingredients can be combined to create great dishes sans calorically dense sauces.

For *Syndrome W* readers, he not only shared several extraordinary recipes for fish, vegetables, and side dishes but also graciously worked with me to decalorize them further.

SUSAN FRITZ, owner, and Peter Milette, chef, Sapphire Restaurant and Oyster Bar

Sapphire Restaurant and Oyster Bar is a longtime favorite of Vail locals and visiting families, with clear appeal for hip snowboarders in their twenties, white-haired seniors, and all manner of diners of ages in between. As Susan Fritz says, "Our food style is simple, fresh, and elegant, maintaining a balance between tradition and innovation, mingling classical technique with ethnic and culinary diversity."

Executive chef and partner Peter Milette incorporates classical European and Asian influences in foods that are healthful and tantalizing.

ALLANA SMITH, dessert and pastry chef, Larkspur

Allana Smith's culinary skills were nurtured by her grandmothers, who taught her the pleasures and treasures of the hearth, especially kuchen, cookies, and candy making. Allana's decision to become a chef followed a one-year stint in Barcelona that brought exposure to new cuisines ("beyond Shake 'n Bake," as she puts it) and the joy of simple rustic fare based on great local produce; she returned home and enrolled in the New England Culinary Institute.

After working with celebrity chefs in restaurants in Chicago, Nantucket, and the Napa Valley, Allana ultimately transitioned from line chef to pastry chef under the tutelage of an alumna from La Varenne.

STEVE TOPPLE, chef de cuisine, Wildflower

I first met Steve Topple in December 2003, seven days after he had taken over as chef de cuisine at Wildflower, one of Vail's premier eateries. I saw that even in his first year, Steve brought a high level of innovation and inspiration to the kitchen; in fact, his energy level is palpable when you walk through the door and the restaurant buzzes with diners' excitement over offerings that change nightly.

Topple's cuisine is always fresh and creative, a clear demonstration of the rule of thumb "less is more," as he intermingles just the barest hint of star anise or chive juice, yet maintains a clean, crisp taste that makes it easy to discern individual elements of his wonderful soups, salads, and entrées.

Steve Topple's enthusiasm for food and for his audience is evident on every visit to Wildflower because he makes a habit of table-hopping to seek feedback on his latest creations. From homemade olive bread to lemon curd tart, his entire menu is sublime, even on the rare nights when Steve is not at the stove and his even younger saucier greets you at your table. As one of his colleagues says, "Steve is a teacher." And that's why I'm pleased to add his lessons to the large classroom of our readers.

REFERENCES

Abbasi, F., V. Kamath, A. A. Rizvi, M. Carantoni, Y. D. Chen, and G. M. Reaven. 1997. Results of a placebo-controlled study of the metabolic effects of the addition of metformin to sulfonylurea-treated patients. Evidence for a central role of adipose tissue. *Diabetes Care* 20 (12): 1863–1869.

Andres, R., D. C. Muller, and J. D. Sorkin. 1993. Long-term effects of change in body weight on all-cause mortality. A review. *Ann Intern Med* 119 (7), Pt. 2: 737–743.

Aronne, L. J. 1998. Modern medical management of obesity: The role of pharmaceutical intervention. *J Am Diet Assoc* 98 (10), Suppl. 2: S23–S26.

———. 2001. Epidemiology, morbidity, and treatment of overweight and obesity. *J Clin Psychiatry* 62, Suppl. 23: 13–22.

Aronne, L. J., and K. R. Segal. 2002. Adiposity and fat distribution outcome measures: Assessment and clinical implications. *Obes Res* 10, Suppl. 1: 14S–21S.

Ayyad, C., and T. Andersen. 2000. Long-term efficacy of dietary treatment of obesity: A systematic review of studies published between 1931 and 1999. *Obes Rev* 1 (2): 113–119.

Blackburn, G. L. 1999. Benefits of weight loss in the treatment of obesity [editorial]. *Am J Clin Nutr* 69 (3): 347–349.

Boden, G., X. Chen, and N. Iqbal. 1998. Acute lowering of plasma fatty acids lowers basal insulin secretion in diabetic and nondiabetic subjects. *Diabetes* 47 (10): 1609–1612.

Bowen, J., M. Noakes, and P. M. Clifton. 2005. Effect of calcium and dairy foods in high protein, energy-restricted diets on weight loss and metabolic parameters in overweight adults. *Int J Obes Relat Metab Disord* 29 (8): 957–965.

Bray, G. A. 2003. Low-carbohydrate diets and realities of weight loss. JAMA 289 (14): 1853–1855.

Bray, G. A., J. C. Lovejoy, S. R. Smith, J. P. DeLany, M. Lefevre, D. Hwang, D. H. Ryan, and D. A. York. 2002. The influence of different fats and fatty acids on obesity, insulin resistance and inflammation. *J Nutr* 132 (9): 2488–2491.

Caan, B., M. Neuhouser, A. Aragaki, et al. 2007. Calcium plus vitamin D supplementation and the risk of postmenopausal weight gain. *Arch Intern Med* 167 (9): 893–902.

Charles, M. A., E. Eschwege, P. Grandmottet, et al. 2000. Treatment with metformin of non-diabetic men with hypertension, hypertriglyceridaemia and central fat distribution: The BIGPRO 1.2 trial. *Diabetes Metab Res Rev* 16 (1): 2–7.

Charles, M. A., P. Morange, E. Eschwege, P. Andre, P. Vague, and I. Vague Juhan. 1998. Effect of weight change and metformin on fibrinolysis and the von Willebrand factor in obese nondiabetic subjects: The BIGPRO1 Study. Biguanides and the prevention of the risk of obesity. *Diabetes Care* 21 (11): 1967–1972.

Cifuentes, M., C. S. Riedt, R. E. Brolin, M. P. Field, R. M. Sherrell, and S. A. Shapses. 2004. Weight loss and calcium intake influence calcium absorption in overweight postmenopausal women. *Am J Clin Nutr* 80 (1): 123–130.

Colditz, G. A., W. C. Willett, A. Rotnitzky, and J. E. Manson. 1995. Weight gain as a risk factor for clinical diabetes mellitus in women. *Ann Intern Med* 122 (7): 481–486.

Conover, C. A., P. D. Lee, J. A. Kanaley, J. T. Clarkson, and M. D. Jensen. 1992. Insulin regulation of insulin-like growth factor binding protein-1 in obese and nonobese humans. *J Clin Endocrinol Metab* 74 (6): 1355–1360.

Davidson, M. B., and A. L. Peters. 1997. An overview of metformin in the treatment of type 2 diabetes mellitus. *Am J Med* 102 (1): 99–110.

DeFronzo, R. A., and E. Ferrannini. 1991. Insulin resistance. A multifaceted syndrome responsible for NIDDM, obesity, hypertension, dyslipidemia, and atherosclerotic cardiovascular disease. *Diabetes Care* 14 (3): 173–194.

Despres, J. P., B. Lamarche, P. Mauriege, B. Cantin, G. R. Dagenais, S. Moorjani, and P. J. Lupien. 1996. Hyperinsulinemia as an independent risk factor for ischemic heart disease. *N Engl J Med* 334 (15): 952–957.

Donahue, R. P., K. Rejman, L. B. Rafalson, J. Dmochowski, S. Stranges, and M. Trevisan. 2007. Sex differences in endothelial function markers before conversion to pre-diabetes: Does the clock start ticking earlier among women? The Western New York Study. *Diabetes Care* 30 (2): 354–359.

Dunn, C. J., and D. H. Peters. 1995. Metformin. A review of its pharmacological properties and therapeutic use in non-insulin-dependent diabetes mellitus. *Drugs* 49 (5): 721–749.

Fontbonne, A. 1994. Why can high insulin levels indicate a risk for coronary heart disease? *Diabetologia* 37 (9): 953–955.

Foster, G. D., H. R. Wyatt, J. O. Hill, et al. 2003. A randomized trial of a low-carbohydrate diet for obesity. *N Engl J Med* 348 (21): 2082–2090.

Foster-Schubert, K. E., J. Overduin, C. E. Prudom, et al. 2008. Acyl and total ghrelin are suppressed strongly by ingested proteins, weakly by lipids, and biphasically by carbohydrates. *J Clin Endocrinol Metab* 93 (5): 1971–1979.

Garber, A. J., J. R. Gavin, and B. J. Goldstein. 1996. Understanding insulin resistance and syndrome X. *Patient Care* (June 15): 198–208.

Gardner, C. D., A. Kiazand, S. Alhassan, et al. 2007. Comparison of the Atkins, Zone, Ornish, and LEARN diets for change in weight and related risk factors among overweight premenopausal women: The A TO Z Weight Loss Study: A randomized trial. *JAMA* 297 (9): 969–977.

Giugliano, D., N. De-Rosa, G. Di-Maro, R. Marfella, R. Acampora, R. Buoninconti, and F. D'Onofrio. 1993. Metformin improves glucose, lipid metabolism, and reduces blood pressure in hypertensive, obese women. *Diabetes Care* 16 (10): 1387–1390.

Goldstein, D. J. 1992. Beneficial health effects of modest weight loss. *Int J Obes Relat Metab Disord* 16 (6): 397–415.

Gregorio, F., F. Ambrosi, P. Filipponi, S. Manfrini, and I. Testa. 1996. Is metformin safe enough for ageing type 2 diabetic patients? *Diabetes Metab* 22 (1): 43–50.

Guven, S., A. El Bershawi, G. E. Sonnenberg, C. R. Wilson, R. G. Hoffmann, G. R. Krakower, and A. H. Kissebah. 1999. Plasma leptin and insulin levels in weight-reduced obese women with normal body mass index: Relationships with body composition and insulin. *Diabetes* 48 (2): 347–352.

Haffner, S. M., and H. Miettinen. 1997. Insulin resistance implications for type II diabetes mellitus and coronary heart disease. *Am J Med* 103 (2): 152–162.

Haffner, S. M., M. P. Stern, H. P. Hazuda, J. A. Pugh, and J. K. Patterson. 1986. Hyperinsulinemia in a population at high risk for non-insulin-dependent diabetes mellitus. *N Engl J Med* 315 (4): 220–224.

Hayes, M. R., C. K. Miller, J. S. Ulbrecht, et al. 2007. A carbohydrate-restricted diet alters gut peptides and adiposity signals in men and women with metabolic syndrome. *J Nutr* 137 (8): 1944–1950.

Helvaci, M. R., H. Kaya, A. Borazan, C. Ozer, M. Seyhanli, and A. Yalcin. 2008. Metformin and parameters of physical health. *Intern Med* 47 (8): 697–703.

Helvaci, M. R., A. Sevinc, C. Camci, and A. Yalcin. 2008. Treatment of white coat hypertension with metformin. *Int Heart J* 49 (6): 671–679.

Hill, J. O., and H. R. Wyatt. 1999. Relapse in obesity treatment: Biology or behavior? [editorial]. *Am J Clin Nutr* 69 (6): 1064–1065.

Howard, B. V., L. Adams-Campbell, C. Allen, et al. 2004. Insulin resistance and weight gain in postmenopausal women of diverse ethnic groups. *Int J Obes Relat Metab Disord* 28 (8): 1039–1047.

Howard, B. V., J. E. Manson, M. L. Stefanick, et al. 2006. Low-fat dietary pattern and weight change over 7 years: The Women's Health Initiative Dietary Modification Trial. *JAMA* 295 (1): 39–49.

Huxley, R., C. M. Lee, F. Barzi, et al. 2009. Coffee, decaffeinated coffee, and tea consumption in relation to incident type 2 diabetes mellitus: A systematic review with meta-analysis. *Arch Intern Med* 169 (22): 2053–2063.

Jakicic, J. M., B. H. Marcus, W. Lang, and C. Janney. 2008. Effect of exercise on 24-month weight loss maintenance in overweight women. *Arch Intern Med* 168 (14): 1550–1559.

Jensen, G. L., M. A. Roy, A. E. Buchanan, and M. B. Berg. 2004. Weight loss intervention for obese older women: Improvements in performance and function. *Obes Res* 12 (11): 1814–1820.

Kassirer, J. P., and M. Angell. 1998. Losing weight—an ill-fated New Year's resolution [editorial; comment]. *N Engl J Med* 338 (1): 52–54.

Knowler, W. C., E. Barrett-Connor, S. E. Fowler, et al. 2002. Reduction in the incidence of type 2 diabetes with lifestyle intervention or metformin. *N Engl J Med* 346 (6): 393–403.

Knowler, W. C., S. E. Fowler, R. F. Hamman, et al. 2009. Ten-year follow-up of diabetes incidence and weight loss in the Diabetes Prevention Program Outcomes Study. *Lancet* 374 (9702): 1677–1686.

Kokkinos, A., C. W. le Roux, K. Alexiadou, et al. 2010. Eating slowly increases the postprandial response of the anorexigenic gut hormones, peptide YY and glucagon-like peptide-1. *J Clin Endocrinol Metab* 95 (1): 333–337.

Korner, J., and L. J. Aronne. 2004. Pharmacological approaches to weight reduction: Therapeutic targets. *J Clin Endocrinol Metab* 89 (6): 2616–2621.

Korner, J., and R. L. Leibel. 2003. To eat or not to eat—how the gut talks to the brain. *N Engl J Med* 349 (10): 926–928.

Kuller, L. H., L. S. Kinzel, K. K. Pettee, et al. 2006. Lifestyle intervention and coronary heart disease risk factor changes over 18 months in postmenopausal women: The Women On the Move through Activity and Nutrition (WOMAN study) clinical trial. *J Women's Health (Larchmt)* 15 (8): 962–974.

Kuller, L. H., A. M. Kriska, L. S. Kinzel, et al. 2007. The clinical trial of Women On the Move through Activity and Nutrition (WOMAN) study. *Contemp Clin Trials* 28 (4): 370–381.

Lee, A., and J. E. Morley. 1998. Metformin decreases food consumption and induces weight loss in subjects with obesity with type II non-insulin-dependent diabetes. *Obes Res* 6 (1): 47–53.

Lee, P. D., C. A. Conover, and D. R. Powell. 1993. Regulation and function of insulin-like growth factor-binding protein-1. *Proc Soc Exp Biol Med* 204 (1): 4–29.

Leibel, R. L. 2002. The role of leptin in the control of body weight. *Nutr Rev* 60 (10), Pt. 2: S15–S19.

Lemne, C., and K. Brismar. 1998. Insulin-like growth factor binding protein-1 as a marker of the metabolic syndrome—a study in borderline hypertension. *Blood Press* 7 (2): 89–95.

Levine, M. D., M. L. Klem, M. A. Kalarchian, et al. 2007. Weight gain prevention among women. *Obesity* 15 (5): 1267–1277.

Liu, S., W. C. Willett, M. J. Stampfer, F. B. Hu, M. Franz, L. Sampson, C. H. Hennekens, and J. E. Manson. 2000. A prospective study of dietary glycemic load, carbohydrate intake, and risk of coronary heart disease in US women. *Am J Clin Nutr* 71 (6): 1455–1461.

Ludwig, D. S., J. A. Majzoub, A. Al Zahrani, G. E. Dallal, I. Blanco, and S. B. Roberts. 1999. High glycemic index foods, overeating, and obesity. *Pediatrics* 103 (3): E26.

Ludwig, D. S., M. A. Pereira, C. H. Kroenke, J. E. Hilner, L. Van-Horn, M. L. Slattery, and D. R. Jacobs Jr. 1999. Dietary fiber, weight gain, and cardiovascular disease risk factors in young adults. *JAMA* 282 (16): 1539–1546.

Malik, V. S., M. B. Schulze, and F. B. Hu. 2006. Intake of sugar-sweetened beverages and weight gain: A systematic review. *Am J Clin Nutr* 84 (2): 274–288.

Manson, J. E., W. C. Willett, M. J. Stampfer, G. A. Colditz, D. J. Hunter, S. E. Hankinson, C. H. Hennekens, and F. E. Speizer. 1995. Body weight and mortality among women. *N Engl J Med* 333 (11): 677–685.

McCarty, M. F. 1998. Utility of metformin as an adjunct to hydroxycitrate/carnitine for reducing body fat in diabetics. *Med Hypotheses* 51 (5): 399–403.

Mogul, H. R., M. Marshall, M. Frey, H. B. Burke, P. S. Wynn, S. Wilker, A. L. Southern, and S. R. Gambert. 1996. Insulin like growth factor-binding protein-1 as a marker for hyperinsulinemia in obese menopausal women. *J Clin Endocrinol Metab* 81 (12): 4492–4495.

Mogul, H. R., S. J. Peterson, B. I. Weinstein, S. Zhang, and A. L. Southren. 2001. Metformin and carbohydrate-modified diet, a novel obesity treatment protocol: Preliminary findings from a case series of non-diabetic women with midlife weight gain and hyperinsulinemia. *Heart Disease* 3 (5): 285–292.

Mogul, H. R., B. Weinstein, and D. Mogul. 1999. Syndrome W: A new model of hyperinsulinemia, hypertension and other CAD risk factors in healthy midlife women with normal glucose (Abstract). *Am J Hypertension* 12 (4): 71A.

Mogul, H. R., B. I. Weinstein, D. B. Mogul, S. J. Peterson, S. Zhang, M. Frey, S. R. Gambert, and A. L. Southren. 2002. Syndrome W: A new model of hyperinsulinemia, hypertension and midlife weight gain in healthy women with normal glucose tolerance. *Heart Dis* 4 (2): 78–85.

Nathan, D. M., M. B. Davidson, R. A. DeFronzo, et al. 2007. Impaired fasting glucose and impaired glucose tolerance: Implications for care. *Diabetes Care* 30 (3): 753–759.

Odeleye, O. E., M. de-Courten, D. J. Pettitt, and E. Ravussin. 1997. Fasting hyperinsulinemia is a predictor of increased body weight gain and obesity in Pima Indian children. *Diabetes* 46 (8): 1341–1345.

Panagiotakos, D. B., C. Pitsavos, C. Chrysohoou, C. Stefanadis, and P. Toutouzas. 2002. The role of traditional Mediterranean type of diet and lifestyle, in the development of acute coronary syndromes: Preliminary results from CARDIO 2000 study. *Cent Eur J Public Health* 10 (1–2): 11–15.

Pi-Sunyer, F. X. 1993. Medical hazards of obesity. *Ann Intern Med* 119 (7), Pt. 2: 655–660.

Pouliot, M. C., J. P. Despres, S. Lemieux, S. Moorjani, C. Bouchard, A. Tremblay, A. Nadeau, and P. J. Lupien. 1994. Waist circumference and abdominal sagittal diameter: Best simple anthropometric indexes of abdominal visceral adipose tissue accumulation and related cardiovascular risk in men and women. *Am J Cardiol* 73 (7): 460–468.

Radak, T. L. 2004. Caloric restriction and calcium's effect on bone metabolism and body composition in overweight and obese premenopausal women. *Nutr Rev* 62 (12): 468–481.

Reaven, G. M. 1988. Banting lecture 1988. Role of insulin resistance in human disease. *Diabetes* 37 (12): 1595–1607.

Rissanen, A. 1998. Pharmacological intervention: The antiobesity approach. *Eur J Clin Invest* 28, Suppl. 2: 27–30.

Rosenbaum, M., E. M. Murphy, S. B. Heymsfield, D. E. Matthews, and R. L. Leibel. 2002. Low-dose leptin administration reverses effects of sustained weight-reduction on energy expenditure and circulating concentrations of thyroid hormones. *J Clin Endocrinol Metab* 87 (5): 2391–2394.

Ruderman, N., D. Chisholm, X. Sunyer Pi, and S. Schneider. 1998. The metabolically obese, normal-weight individual revisited. *Diabetes* 47 (5): 699–713.

Sacks, F. M., G. A. Bray, V. J. Carey, et al. 2009. Comparison of weight-loss diets with different compositions of fat, protein, and carbohydrates. *N Engl J Med* 360 (9): 859–873.

Salmeron, J., J. E. Manson, M. J. Stampfer, G. A. Colditz, A. L. Wing, and W. C. Willett. 1997. Dietary fiber, glycemic load, and risk of non-insulin-dependent diabetes mellitus in women. *JAMA* 277 (6): 472–477.

Salonen, J. T., T. A. Lakka, H. M. Lakka, V. P. Valkonen, S. A. Everson, and G. A. Kaplan. 1998. Hyperinsulinemia is associated with the incidence of hypertension and dyslipidemia in middle-aged men. *Diabetes* 47 (2): 270–275.

Salpeter, S. R., N. S. Buckley, J. A. Kahn, and E. E. Salpeter. 2008. Meta-analysis: Metformin treatment in persons at risk for diabetes mellitus. *Am J Med* 121 (2): 149–157.

Sbrocco, T., R. C. Nedegaard, J. M. Stone, and E. L. Lewis. 1999. Behavioral choice treatment promotes continuing weight loss: Preliminary results of a cognitive-behavioral decision-based treatment for obesity. *J Consult Clin Psychol* 67 (2): 260–266.

Schwartz, M. W., S. C. Woods, R. J. Seeley, G. S. Barsh, D. G. Baskin, and R. L. Leibel. 2003. Is the energy homeostasis system inherently biased toward weight gain? *Diabetes* 52 (2): 232–238.

Serdula, M. K., A. H. Mokdad, D. F. Williamson, D. A. Galuska, J. M. Mendlein, and G. W. Heath. 1999. Prevalence of attempting weight loss and strategies for controlling weight. *JAMA* 282 (14): 1353–1358.

Shai, I., D. Schwarzfuchs, Y. Henkin, et al. 2008. Weight loss with a low-carbohydrate, Mediterranean, or low-fat diet. *N Engl J Med* 359 (3): 229–241.

Shintani, M., Y. Ogawa, K. Ebihara, et al. 2001. Ghrelin, an endogenous growth hormone secretagogue, is a novel orexigenic peptide that antagonizes leptin action through the activation of hypothalamic neuropeptide Y/Y1 receptor pathway. *Diabetes* 50 (2): 227–232.

Skov, A. R., S. Toubro, B. Ronn, L. Holm, and A. Astrup. 1999. Randomized trial on protein vs. carbohydrate in ad libitum fat reduced diet for the treatment of obesity. *Int J Obes* 23:529–536.

Speechly, D. P., and R. Buffenstein. 2000. Appetite dysfunction in obese males: Evidence for role of hyperinsulinaemia in passive overconsumption with a high fat diet. *Eur J Clin Nutr* 54 (3): 225–233.

Spieth, L. E., J. D. Harnish, C. M. Lenders, L. B. Raezer, M. A. Pereira, S. J. Hangen, and D. S. Ludwig. 2000. A low-glycemic index diet in the treatment of pediatric obesity. *Arch Pediatr Adolesc Med* 154 (9): 947–951.

Stern, M. P. 1996. Do non-insulin-dependent diabetes mellitus and cardiovascular disease share common antecedents? *Ann Intern Med* 124 (1), Pt. 2: 110–116.

Stout, R. W. 1996. Hyperinsulinemia and atherosclerosis. *Diabetes* 45, Suppl. 3: S45–S46.

Suikkari, A. M., V. A. Koivisto, E. M. Rutanen, Jarvinen H. Yki, S. L. Karonen, and M. Seppala. 1988. Insulin regulates the serum levels of low molecular weight insulin-like growth factor-binding protein. *J Clin Endocrinol Metab* 66 (2): 266–272.

Sulkin, T. V., D. Bosman, and A. J. Krentz. 1997. Contraindications to metformin therapy in patients with NIDDM. *Diabetes Care* 20 (6): 925–928.

Sun, Q., M. K. Townsend, O. I. Okereke, O. H. Franco, F. B. Hu, and F. Grodstein. 2009. Adiposity and weight change in mid-life in relation to healthy survival after age 70 in women: Prospective cohort study. *BMJ* 339:b3796.

Suzuki, M., M. Ikebuchi, K. Shinozaki, Y. Hara, M. Tsushima, T. Matsuyama, and Y. Harano. 1996. Mechanism and clinical implication of insulin resistance syndrome. *Diabetes* 45, Suppl. 3: S52–S54.

Tchernof, A., and E. T. Poehlman. 1998. Effects of the menopause transition on body fatness and body fat distribution. *Obesity Research* 6 (3): 246–254.

Travers, S. H., J. I. Labarta, S. E. Gargosky, R. G. Rosenfeld, B. W. Jeffers, and R. H. Eckel. 1998. Insulin-like growth factor binding protein-I levels are strongly associated with insulin sensitivity and obesity in early pubertal children. *J Clin Endocrinol Metab* 83 (6): 1935–1939.

Willett, W. C., and R. L. Leibel. 2002. Dietary fat is not a major determinant of body fat. *Am J Med* 113, Suppl. 9B: 47S–59S.

Wing, R. R., M. G. Goldstein, K. J. Acton, L. L. Birch, J. M. Jakicic, J. F. Sallis Jr., D. Smith-West, R. W. Jeffery, and R. S. Surwit. 2001. Behavioral science research in diabetes: Lifestyle changes related to obesity, eating behavior, and physical activity. *Diabetes Care* 24 (1): 117–123.

Wing, R. R., K. A. Matthews, L. H. Kuller, D. Smith, D. Becker, P. L. Plantinga, and E. N. Meilahn. 1992. Environmental and familial contributions to insulin levels and change in insulin levels in middle-aged women. *JAMA* 268 (14): 1890–1895.

Wolever, T. M., D. J. Jenkins, A. L. Jenkins, and R. G. Josse. 1991. The glycemic index: Methodology and clinical implications. *Am J Clin Nutr* 54 (5): 846–854.

Wylie-Rosett, J., C. Swencionis, A. Caban, A. Friedler, and N. Schaffer. 1997. *The complete weight loss workbook.* Alexandria, VA: American Diabetes Association.

Yanovski, Jack A., and Susan Z. Yanovski. 2003. Treatment of pediatric and adolescent obesity. *JAMA* 289 (14): 1851.

Zemel, M. B. 2004. Role of calcium and dairy products in energy partitioning and weight management. *Am J Clin Nutr* 79 (5): 907S–912S.

———. 2005. Calcium and dairy modulation of obesity risk. *Obes Res* 13 (1): 192–193.

Zemel, M. B., W. Thompson, A. Milstead, K. Morris, and P. Campbell. 2004. Calcium and dairy acceleration of weight and fat loss during energy restriction in obese adults. *Obes Res* 12 (4): 582–590.

INDEX

ABOUT THE AUTHOR

Epidemiologist, endocrinologist, and author, **Harriette Mogul**, M.D., M.P.H., first identified and described Syndrome W and garnered page-one headlines in *Internal Medicine News*, the monthly newspaper of internists in America, following her first scientific presentation of this common but previously overlooked female phenomenon.

A graduate of Bryn Mawr College, the Albert Einstein College of Medicine, and the Columbia School of Public Health, Dr. Mogul was an early pioneer in women's health research. While director of Student Health Services at Barnard College, she founded the Barnard-Columbia Institute for Medical Research in Women and spearheaded some of the first large national studies on women and weight more than twenty years ago. After returning to full-time academic medicine, she went on to complete a fellowship in endocrinology and metabolism at Westchester Medical Center and to initiate laboratory and clinical studies of women who were at other and older stages of the life cycle.

Today Dr. Mogul serves as associate professor and director of research in the Division of Endocrinology at New York Medical College. For the past ten years, the focus of her research and clinical practice has been the menopausal transition, obesity, and disorders of insulin resistance and growth hormone deficiency in adults. Dr. Mogul's perspectives on estrogen use in menopause have been highlighted in *Time* magazine and the *New York Times*. Publication "firsts" include the description of a simple blood test for insulin abnormalities in nondiabetic women; the definition of a disorder of weight gain and insulin resistance in nondiabetic, menopausal women—Syndrome W; and the use of metformin, a widely used diabetes medication, to treat obesity in women with normal blood sugar levels. This publication has been cited in Reuters, the *New York Times*, and the *Wall Street Journal*.

Living in Chappaqua, New York, Dr. Mogul is the wife of Malcolm D. Mogul and the mother of Jennifer Mogul, M.D., a child and adolescent psychiatrist; Fred Mogul of WNYC; and Douglas Mogul, M.D., M.P.H., currently a fellow in pediatric gastroenterology at Johns Hopkins Medical Center.